Praise for
Overcoming Postpartum Depression and Anxiety

"A well-researched, compassionate book that explains the types of mental health problems women may develop during pregnancy and after delivery. The book's comprehensive treatment information will be helpful to both women suffering from postpartum psychiatric disorders and to healthcare providers who treat them."

Catherine Cram, M.S., Author
Exercising Through Your Pregnancy

"I highly recommend this book to anyone dealing with a perinatal mood disorder. Well organized and easy to understand, the book lays out the range of symptoms, possible causes, and treatment options. It's a wonderful book!"

Ann Smith, R.N., C.N.M.
President, Postpartum Support International

"I felt great during my pregnancy, but after the birth of my child forty-six years ago, I felt so detached, and I avoided the baby. I thought I was a bad mother. I now realize I was depressed. This was back in the 1970s, and postpartum depression was so often not diagnosed or treated. How I wish I'd had this book then."

Arlene, 67

"I found the first edition of *Overcoming Postpartum Depression and Anxiety* invaluable in my work with women who were suffering with postpartum psychiatric disorders. The book has been so helpful to them. I believe this updated edition will be even more helpful to my clients and their families."

Canda Byrne, D.N.P
Associate Professor, University of Pikeville
Pikeville, Kentucky

"A user-friendly book, packed full of useful information about the types of perinatal psychiatric disorders and how they are treated. The women's real-life stories about their mood disorders bring the book to life!"

Susanne Somerville, Clinical Psychologist
King Edward Memorial Hospital
Western Australia

Overcoming Postpartum Depression & Anxiety

Third Edition

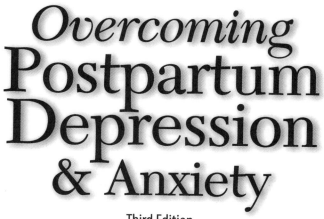

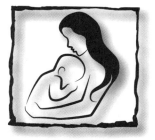

LINDA SEBASTIAN, A.R.N.P.

Addicus Books
Omaha, Nebraska

An Addicus Nonfiction Book

ISBN 978-1-943886-00-5

Cover and typography by Jack Kusler

This book is not intended to serve as a substitute for a physician. Nor is it the author's intent to give medical advice contrary to that of an attending physician.

Library of Congress Cataloging-in-Publication Data

Names: Sebastian, Linda,—author.
Title: Overcoming postpartum depression and anxiety / Linda Sebastian, A.R.N.P.
Description: Third edition. | Omaha, Nebraska : Addicus Books, Inc., [2016] | Includes bibliographical references and index.
Identifiers: LCCN 2016012872 (print) | LCCN 2016015980 (ebook) | ISBN 9781943886005 (paperback) | ISBN 9781943886425 (PDF) | ISBN 9781943886449 (MOBI) | ISBN 9781943886432 (EPUB)
Subjects: LCSH: Postpartum depression. | Anxiety in women. | BISAC: HEALTH & FITNESS / Women's Health. | SELF-HELP / Depression.
Classification: LCC RG852 .S43 2016 (print) | LCC RG852 (ebook) | DDC 618.7/6—dc23
LC record available at https://lccn.loc.gov/2016012872

Addicus Books, Inc.
P.O. Box 45327
Omaha, Nebraska 68145
www.AddicusBooks.com
Printed in the United States of America
10 9 8 7 6 5 4 3 2 1

*To all the women and their families
with whom I've had the privilege of working*

Contents

Acknowledgments

A special thanks to the many people who helped make this third edition happen: Ann Smith, nurse midwife and president of Postpartum Support International, and Cheryl Beck, Ph.D. Deep gratitude to Peg Walsh for her encouragement. I thank Dr. Steve Machlin for his support. And a special thank you to Rene Almeling for the research help. And for my husband Guy—many, many thanks for your encouragement. I appreciate this more than you can know.

I also wish to thank those who have helped me with previous editions of this book. I extend special thanks to Tom Averill; Meredith Titus, Ph.D.; Elizabeth Davis; Jeff Ostergren; and especially Canda Byrne, A.R.N.P., who hung in there with me from start to finish. Thanks to Lee Cohen, M.D., for his pioneering work in the field of perinatal psychiatry and for his encouragement, and Martin Maldonado, M.D.; Robert Barnett, M.D.; Grace Morrison, M.D.; and Breck Edds, M.D., for sharing their perspectives and contributing to this book.

I thank Manya Schmidt, C.N.M., A.R.N.P, for her contributions and her guidance, and Joyce Venis, R.N., of *Depression after Delivery* for her contributions. I am also grateful to the Menninger Writers Group for their helpful comments, encouragement, and, especially, writing comradeship. A special thanks goes to Mary Ann Clifft, director of scientific publications at Menninger, for her guidance and editing. To Kathryn Zerbe, M.D.; Harriet Lerner, Ph.D.; and Glen Gabbard, M.D., many thanks for sharing your wisdom. To the staff at the Professional Library at the Menninger Foundation, your help was invaluable to me.

Introduction

Like most new mothers or mothers-to-be, you probably have heard of postpartum depression. You probably thought that it was something that happens to other women, but would never happen to you. That's what I thought, too. During my first pregnancy, I thought motherhood would be a blissful and perfect time. After the birth of my first child, I found myself crying for no reason several times a day. Irritable and cranky, I often found myself in tears over the slightest problem. Because I couldn't understand why I was crying, I was constantly worried. I felt totally inadequate as a mother. I felt both shame and fear that I was not going to be able to cope with this new little person in my life. The thoughts overwhelmed me.

I had read several books about pregnancy and becoming a new mother, but I had not read anything to make me imagine that I would experience the emotional turmoil that I was having. After all, I had wanted a baby very much. But, even though I thought I was prepared for motherhood, I was caught off guard by the roller coaster of my moods. This scary time lasted two weeks before I began to feel better.

Fortunately, I had an understanding and helpful partner who took over the care of our baby when he got home at night so I could rest. I felt very guilty and thought I was letting my husband down by not being a better mother for our new baby. A neighbor who had several children helped me through this time by assuring me that I was not going crazy, and that I would recover. Her advice was simple: get as much sleep as you can and ask friends and family not to visit for a while. She didn't tell me not to cry or ask me why I was crying. This kind neighbor's support was so helpful, I don't know what I would have done without her.

In hindsight, I realize I had postpartum blues. Now, my "baby" is almost forty. Yet very little has changed in the way of public awareness of postpartum depression. Our society does not adequately prepare new mothers and their partners for the overwhelming adjustment to parenthood. The childbirth classes we took emphasized only how to prepare for the big event: labor and delivery. We learned all about breathing and stages of labor. But there was little discussion about the adjustment period following the birth and no mention of how devastating postpartum blues can be, let alone the possibility of more severe depression. The mind-set that mothers blissfully enjoy being mothers from day one only increases the risk of emotional problems for some women. Tens of thousands of women are simply not prepared for postpartum psychiatric disorders.

As a nurse practitioner, I have worked with women who experienced unexpected mood changes or uncomfortable tension after the birth of their babies. I have seen many women and their families suffer from the effects of depression and anxiety. The lack of information available only worsens the situation. Often, neither health care professionals nor the public have ready access to information about the emotional problems that may occur after childbirth. As you will read, there are many reasons for this lack of information.

When I wrote the first edition of this book, published in 1998, I had no idea the book would be so useful for so many people. Now, almost twenty years later, I am amazed by the amount of research and information that has added to our knowledge base about the psychiatric problems that are the most common complication of pregnancy and childbirth. Today, we know far more about the prevention of and the cultural aspects of perinatal psychiatric disorders. Treatment is now more definitive, and there are more non-medication options available. Changes in diagnostic categories have helped clinicians identify and treat problems, especially in the area of post-traumatic stress disorders and obsessive-compulsive disorders, both during pregnancy and after giving birth. Research is also

Introduction

underway to identify the role genetics may play in the development of psychiatric disorders in women who are pregnant or have just given birth. Unfortunately, what has not changed is the toll that psychiatric illness takes on new mothers, their babies, and their families going through this trauma. There is still a great deal of stigma (and ignorance) in our society about mental health problems; even some health care professionals are uninformed about postpartum psychiatric disorders. But progress is being made, and it is exciting to realize that the care of women and their families has improved in recent years and will, hopefully, continue to do so.

I wrote this book for women who are experiencing mood changes or anxiety during pregnancy or after delivery. It is my hope that the book will provide you with the kind of information that would have been helpful to me when, as a new mother, I thought I was going crazy, and I felt all alone. Learning about postpartum depression and anxiety is your first step in understanding what may be happening to you. As you will come to understand, having emotional problems during or after pregnancy does not mean you are weak. It does not mean you're a bad mother, and perhaps most importantly, you are not alone.

1

Postpartum Disorders:
An Overview

I was so excited about having baby. We had waited four years after we were married and saved our money, so I didn't have to go back to work. I worried about the baby having all its parts or being healthy, but I didn't worry about me. When I couldn't stop crying after I got home with the baby, I was so scared and thought I was a terrible mother. No one told me this might happen.

Annette, 32-year-old mother

Annette's anticipation of the birth of her child is common. Most women expect an uneventful pregnancy and delivery. If anything, women usually worry more about the health of their babies than about their own health. For the majority of women, this time in their lives is, indeed, a time of health, happiness, and well-being. However, many women experience problems with depression and anxiety both during their pregnancy and after delivery.

Because so many woman are not aware of potential emotional complications after childbirth, those who do have these problems often feel alone and isolated. This can have devastating consequences for the woman and her baby, and their relationship. Often, women assume that if they are depressed or anxious after the birth of a baby, it means they are not good mothers.

Starting the Journey of Discovery

If you are pregnant or a new mother, it is important that you and your family learn about symptoms that describe what you may be experiencing emotionally. For some women, it is

1

a relief to know that there are medical reasons why they may feel anxious or depressed. You will also realize that you are not alone. Hundreds of thousands of other woman experience overwhelming and frightening feelings before, during, or after their pregnancies. This book is intended to explain the basics of postpartum depression and to provide guidance to help you cope and recover.

What Is Postpartum Depression?

Postpartum depression is a mood disorder that occurs in mothers after the birth of their babies. Sometimes, the depression starts during delivery, but for many women, the first weeks after delivery marks the beginning of a depression. Between 10 and 20 percent of women who have a baby will have some form of psychiatric symptoms, including depression. Postpartum depression is a term that includes a spectrum of problems, including *postpartum blues* on the mild end of the spectrum to the more severe end of the spectrum that includes *postpartum depression* (a major depression), *postpartum anxiety,* and *postpartum psychosis.* We'll examine an overview of each of these conditions in this chapter.

There is a strong connection between anxiety and depression. Just as most women who suffer from major depression also have some anxiety, women with anxiety disorders often experience some depression. Usually these problems occur together. In fact, one study found that a previous history of an anxiety disorder was a bigger risk factor for postpartum disorders than a previous episode of depression. Anxiety disorders are covered separately in chapter 4 to help you clearly understand the symptoms.

Because postpartum mood and anxiety disorders have different symptoms, different treatments, and possibly different causes, each one will be discussed separately in this book. Bear in mind, however, that sometimes the problems overlap and may be difficult to distinguish from one another. For example, in the second or third week postpartum, it may be difficult to tell if you are experiencing postpartum blues or postpartum depression. For this reason, it is important to consult a mental health professional as soon as you notice problems.

Understanding Terms

The term *postpartum depression* is often used to describe any psychiatric problem a pregnant or postpartum woman (one who has given birth) may have, even though actual depression may not be one of her symptoms. The unclear terms used for the various disorders adds to the confusion for much of the public as well as for some professionals. This means that women with depression or anxiety are often overlooked or are not seen as having significant problems. Clinicians know that anxiety disorders are common for pregnant and postpartum women; however, because these problems are not always recognized, some new mothers often go untreated.

In this book, I will use the specific terms *postpartum blues, postpartum depression, postpartum psychosis,* and *postpartum anxiety.* However, for the sake of clarity I will often use the more general term *postpartum depression* even though that term may not be the official clinical term for the problem being discussed.

Today, clinicians and researchers are beginning to use a new term—*perinatal psychiatric disorders.* (*Perinatal* refers to the time just before or after the birth of a baby.) This term represents the understanding that many of the problems with mood and anxiety we see in the postpartum period actually begin during pregnancy. Perinatal psychiatry is a subspecialty in the field of psychiatry that began emerging in the early 1990s.

Types of Postpartum Disorders

Let's examine the various types of postpartum disorders to better understand the levels of depression a woman may experience. Each of these conditions will be examined more thoroughly in later chapters.

Baby Blues

The term *baby blues* refers to a brief time of temporary tearfulness, mood swings, fatigue, and perhaps irritability that typically lasts only one to two weeks after childbirth. This is common after giving birth and bringing a baby home. The baby blues usually resolve without treatment. But while they last, it is upsetting for the new mother and her family.

3

Postpartum Depression

Postpartum depression refers to a state of major depression in which one's mood is marked by feelings of guilt, sadness, lack of enjoyment, fatigue, and problems in concentration. More severe symptoms may include thoughts of harming yourself or your baby.

Bipolar Disorder

This mood disorder is characterized by fluctuating moods. There are episodes of depression at times and then there may be periods of excessive energy and grandiose thinking. Other symptoms of bipolar disorder may include irritability, impulsivity, and poor judgment.

Anxiety Disorders

Several kinds of *anxiety disorders* can occur during and after pregnancy. Anxiety disorders include a spectrum of fearful states. These disorders range from excessive and uncontrollable worry in *generalized anxiety disorder,* to symptoms such as a racing heart, shortness of breath, and episodes of fear in *panic attacks.*

Postpartum Psychosis

Psychosis is a state of confusion, agitation, being out of touch with reality, and having delusions (false beliefs) and/or hallucinations (seeing things or hearing things that are non-existent). For example, a new mother may hear voices telling her to kill her baby; or the voices may convince her that the baby is possessed or is a demon. Postpartum psychosis is considered a psychiatric emergency because of the risk of harm to the baby and the mother. This condition usually develops within the first few days after delivery.

Post-Traumatic Stress Disorder

Post-traumatic stress disorder (PTSD) is a specific kind of anxiety disorder marked by re-experiencing a trauma such as a health scare for the pregnant mother or her fears about the health of the fetus. She may also have nightmares and wish to avoid any situations that provoke unwanted thoughts or feelings. With post-traumatic stress disorder, these symptoms do not lessen in intensity over time. It is becoming apparent that this condition is more common than was previously known, and can have long-lasting consequences for the mother and baby.

Obsessive-Compulsive Disorder (OCD)

This disorder is often overlooked but is actually quite common in the postpartum period. *Obsessions* are repetitive intrusive thoughts, and *compulsions* are repetitive behaviors that are accompanied by feelings of guilt and shame. A woman suffering from OCD is unable to stop the thoughts and behaviors and sometimes has difficulty taking care of her baby.

Causes of Postpartum Disorders

Clinicians and researchers still do not know why some women will have psychiatric problems during pregnancy and after delivery while others will not. There is ongoing research about genetic predisposition and the role of stress, but not all women are affected in the same way. Many people assume hormones are the culprit. However, all women experience the same hormonal shifts during pregnancy and after delivery, but not all women get depressed or anxious.

Causes of specific postpartum disorders will be discussed in more depth in later chapters. Although the causes of these disorders are not completely clear, there is considerable research about the risk factors that may predict who will develop problems.

Each disorder described in this book has a unique set of symptoms that are used for reaching a diagnosis; the symptoms for each type of disorder will be explained in subsequent chapters.

Risk Factors for Postpartum Disorders

Even though clinicians and researchers are unable to pinpoint an exact cause of every case of postpartum disorder, they have been able to identify factors that are known to put women as risk for postpartum problems.

Previous Episode of Depression or Anxiety

If a woman has previously suffered depression after childbirth or has had other episodes of depression or anxiety in her lifetime, she is among those most likely to develop problems with the birth of a child and perhaps during pregnancy. She is also at risk if she has experienced severe postpartum blues or has had mood changes related to her menstrual cycle.

Researchers in Italy conducted a fairly large study of 600 pregnant women to see if *panic disorder* (a specific type of anxiety marked by episodes of panic or fear of death) was a strong predictor of postpartum depression. They found that of all the anxiety disorders, panic disorder or even a family history of panic disorder was a strong predictor of mood disorders after the birth of a baby.

Major Stress Resulting from Change

Another risk factor is major stress or change during pregnancy. Even a positive change such as a move to a new house may place more emotional burden on a pregnant woman. Other stressors, such as a death in the family, conflict with a spouse or partner, and even financial stress, can have an adverse effect on the new mother.

A Mother's Health Concerns for Herself or Her Baby

Problems with the mother's health during pregnancy and delivery are a significant risk factor for postpartum problems. These problems range from a mother's fears of elevated blood pressure to concerns about becoming anemic. (If you're anemic during pregnancy, your red blood cells may not be delivering enough oxygen to your tissues and the baby.) Other stressors a pregnant woman may find herself facing are concerns about the health of the baby before and during delivery. For example, during delivery, a newborn's heart rate is constantly monitored; if there are irregularities in the baby's heart rate, it is an issue that will be of concern to medical staff. If there has been a "scare" during delivery, it is not uncommon for a new mother to have nightmares about the baby having health problems even after the baby has arrived and is doing well.

Lack of Emotional Support

A non-supportive spouse or partner may make the new mother at more risk for developing depression. If family members are not supportive or helpful, the new mother may feel isolated. Also, the time at home after a baby is born may lead a new mother to be more socially isolated, especially if she worked outside the home before delivery. Further, if the new mother is not well acquainted with neighbors, she'll lack close-by emotional support.

Childhood Abuse and Trauma

Two significant risk factors for depression in general, not only during pregnancy and postpartum, are childhood abuse and trauma. Sexual abuse, physical abuse, neglect, and overwhelming traumatic experiences such as the loss of a parent or sibling place women at risk for depression and anxiety even without the added stress of pregnancy and motherhood. Previous abuse and trauma that has not been addressed may become more prominent during this time of major change in a woman's life as she becomes a new mother.

Premature Birth

According to studies in multiple cultures, a premature birth increases the risk for postpartum depression significantly. *Premature birth,* also known as *preterm birth,* occurs when a baby is born before thirty-seven weeks of pregnancy. Preterm birth is the greatest contributor to infant death.

Preterm birth in the United States occurs in one out of ten deliveries—about 10 percent. It is much higher in some countries, such as Pakistan, where the preterm birth rate is as high as 15 percent, and it is lower in Europe, at 6 percent.

Previous Pregnancy Loss

Although a previous pregnancy loss is known to be a risk factor for developing symptoms of postpartum disorders, the impact on women who have experienced more than one pregnancy loss seems to be even greater. According to some researchers, recurrent pregnancy loss can adversely affect up to 3 percent of women wanting to have a child.

Partner Violence

Thirty-seven studies looked at intimate partner violence as a risk factor for postpartum disorders. Researchers found that exposure to partner violence increased the risk for *major depression* in women two- to threefold. And the increase for postpartum depression was one and one-half- to twofold. Spouse or partner abuse is a risk factor for a woman to experience depression at any stage of life, so this is not a surprising finding.

Other Risk Factors

A longtime nurse researcher in the field of perinatal psychiatry, Cheryl Beck, Ph.D., conducted an analysis of eighty-four studies to further examine risk factors. In addition to the risk factors mentioned above, Dr. Beck discovered that an unplanned pregnancy may put a woman at risk for mood changes. Dr. Beck also found infant temperament, such as a difficult-to-soothe baby, may be a major stressor for the mother. Poor-quality child care, or the lack of child care, can negatively impact the mother's mental health. Marital status, such as being unmarried even if the relationship is stable, may influence a women's mood or anxiety during pregnancy or after delivery.

Predicting Who's at Risk

It is helpful to detect problems with mood or anxiety as early as possible in order to begin treatment or perhaps provide resources to help prevent problems. If women, their families, and clinicians know the risk factors and address the problems early in the pregnancy, they can attempt to lessen the severity of or even possibly prevent the illness.

Being aware of risk factors is important because of the frequency of postpartum psychiatric problems. Sixty to 80 percent of all women who bear children experience milder problems such as postpartum blues, and about 10 to 20 percent will develop major depression or severe anxiety. Only 1 percent develop the more severe psychotic depression.

To detect women at risk for postpartum depression and anxiety, and refer them to appropriate psychiatric professionals, obstetricians and nurse midwives will ask pregnant women a few questions about their mental health history. Questions about the stress levels in the woman's life—especially about the quality of her marital relationship—are just as important as questions about physical symptoms. Lisa's story attests to this:

I was told I was at risk and was referred to a therapist in my third trimester. I was so relieved to have someone recognize that I needed psychological help as well as monitoring of my pregnancy. Things went much better because I had emotional help and support.

8

Postpartum Disorders: An Overview

One tool that has been used for many years by clinicians and researchers for screening for postpartum disorders is the Edinburgh Postnatal Depression Scale, shown below.

You may wish to answer the questions and then follow the scoring directions at the end of the questionnaire. *Important note:* this questionnaire is a screening tool only. Do not use it to diagnose yourself. It is an indicator of depression and does not detect anxiety. Answer the questions based on how you have felt the past week.

Edinburgh Postnatal Depression Scale (EPDS)

Name:_____

Address:_____

Your Date of Birth:_____

Your Baby's Date of Birth_____

Phone:_____

As you are pregnant or have recently had a baby, we would like to know how you are feeling. Please check the answer that comes closest to how you have felt IN THE PAST 7 DAYS, not just how you feel today.

Here is an example.

I have felt happy:
☐   Yes, all the time
☑   Yes, most of the time
    This would mean: "I have felt happy most of the time" during the past week.
    Please complete the other questions in the same way.
☐   No, not very often
☐   No, not at all

In the past 7 days:

1. I have been able to laugh and see the funny side of things.
☐   As much as I always could **(0)**
☐   Not quite so much now **(1)**
☐   Definitely not so much now **(2)**
☐   Not at all **(3)**

2. I have looked forward with enjoyment to things.
☐   As much as I ever did **(0)**
☐   Rather less than I used to **(1)**
☐   Definitely less than I used to **(2)**
☐   Hardly at all **(3)**

Edinburgh Postnatal Depression Scale (EPDS) (Continued)

3. I have blamed myself unnecessarily when things went wrong.
- ☐ Yes, most of the time (3)
- ☐ Yes, some of the time (2)
- ☐ Not very often (1)
- ☐ No, never (0)

4. I have been anxious or worried for no good reason.
- ☐ No, not at all (0)
- ☐ Hardly ever (1)
- ☐ Yes, sometimes (2)
- ☐ Yes, very often (3)

5. I have felt scared or panicky for no very good reason.
- ☐ Yes, quite a lot (3)
- ☐ Yes, sometimes (2)
- ☐ No, not much (1)
- ☐ No, not at all (0)

6. Things have been bothering me.
- ☐ Yes, most of the time I haven't been able to cope at all (3)
- ☐ Yes, sometimes I haven't been coping as well as usual (2)
- ☐ No, most of the time I have coped quite well (1)
- ☐ No, I have been coping as well as ever (0)

7. I have been so unhappy that I have had difficulty sleeping.
- ☐ Yes, most of the time (3)
- ☐ Yes, sometimes (2)
- ☐ Not very often (1)
- ☐ No, not at all (0)

8. I have felt sad or miserable.
- ☐ Yes, most of the time (3)
- ☐ Yes, quite often (2)
- ☐ Not very often (1)
- ☐ No, not at all (0)

9. I have been so unhappy that I have been crying.
- ☐ Yes, most of the time (3)
- ☐ Yes, quite often (2)
- ☐ Only occasionally (1)
- ☐ No, never (0)

Edinburgh Postnatal Depression Scale (EPDS) (Continued)

10. The thought of harming myself has occurred to me.
- ☐ Yes, quite often (3)
- ☐ Sometimes (2)
- ☐ Hardly ever (1)
- ☐ Never (0)

Edinburgh Source: Cox, J.L.,Holden, J.M., and Sagovsky, R. 1987. Detection of postnatal depression: Development of the 10-item Edinburgh Postnatal Depression Scale. British Journal of Psychiatry 150:782-786 . 2 Source: K. L. Wisner, B. L. Parry, C. M. Piontek, Postpartum Depression N Engl J Med Vol. 347, No 3, July 18,2002, 194-199

Scoring the Edinburgh Scale

After answering the questions, go back and add up the numbers that appear in parenthesis next to each of your answers. A score of ten or higher indicates depression. If you answered "yes" to the last question about harming yourself, you should contact your physician or clinician immediately.

Diagnosis and Treatment of Postpartum Depression and Anxiety

With the exception of specific screening tools such as the Edinburgh Postnatal Depression Scale, postpartum disorders are diagnosed using the same tools and tests used for other psychiatric disorders. A screening tool for anxiety will be discussed in chapter 4.

Treatment consists of a variety of interventions, including medication and psychotherapy; supportive measures, such as increased rest and nutrition; and, sometimes, hospitalization may be used, depending on the severity of the illness.

Why Postpartum Disorders Are Underdiagnosed

Many women still are not informed that they may have mood or anxiety problems after delivery. And many families simply do not understand psychiatric problems and treatment. Additionally, unfortunately, many people in our society still have a negative and shaming view of people with mental health concerns. Following are a number of factors that contribute to the lack of awareness about postpartum problems.

Lack of Experience with Babies

In today's smaller families, new mothers often have had little previous experience caring for babies of others or being around women who are having babies. A new mother's lack of experience, coupled with unrealistic expectations, increases her fear of inadequacy. Many women have never been aware of anyone else who has had depression or anxiety after delivery. Because of the perceived stigma that may accompany postpartum disorders, many women do not tell other women what has happened to them. This contributes to the lack of information about risk factors for postpartum problems.

Lack of Family Help and Support

Many extended families live too far away to help a new mother at home during the crucial first two weeks after delivery. Many working women who give birth feel alone because both their peer and social groups or their families are unavailable. Having a baby separates a woman from her normal support system and keeps her isolated. Such isolation may contribute to mood disorders.

Society's Expectation for the "Good Mother"

Culturally, our society pays little attention to women and their partners during pregnancy and delivery. There is an expectation that all will be well after delivery. The mother should go home to do what comes naturally: take care of her baby without help or guidance. However, more attention should be paid not only to the new mother and her mental health, but to the father as well because we now know he is also at risk for developing depression and anxiety. New research on the topic of fathers' depression will be discussed in chapter 9. The postpartum period is the time of highest risk in a woman's lifetime to be hospitalized with a psychiatric disorder. This is not a trivial issue that should be ignored.

Health Professionals' Lack of Knowledge

Compounding the confusion for new mothers and their families is health care professionals' general lack of awareness about postpartum disorders. Many of the major obstetric and gynecologic texts in use today generally do not mention the risk of postpartum mood disorders. As a result of this omission, many nurses and physicians do not recognize perinatal psychiatric disorders; they are not consistently assessing women for mood disorders during pregnancy or after delivery.

Postpartum Disorders: An Overview

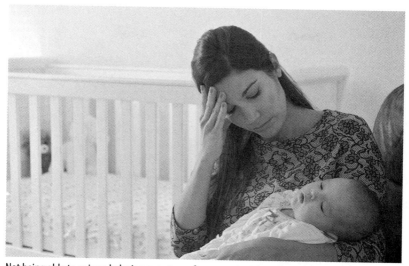

Not being able to enjoy a baby is a symptom of many perinatal psychiatric disorders.

Fortunately, this oversight seems to be changing. Steve Machlin, M.D., a psychiatrist in private practice for more than twenty years, has treated many pregnant and postpartum women for mood and anxiety disorders. Dr. Machlin states: "I don't think I had any lectures on perinatal psychiatric problems during medical school, but when I go to conferences and continuing education meetings now, the programs about perinatal psychiatric problems are well attended. I think there is more interest and more awareness about these problems."

Anxiety and depression in the postpartum period are among the few psychiatric disorders for which mental health professionals have been successful in identifying risk factors. This has enabled them to treat problems earlier and perhaps modify the severity of symptoms.

However, there is still debate as to whether postpartum disorders are unique to this time period after giving birth or are similar to depression and anxiety found in both men and women at other times in their lives. In one British study, women who had gynecologic surgery were compared to women who had just delivered a baby. A questionnaire examined their mood changes. The researchers found that there were signifi-

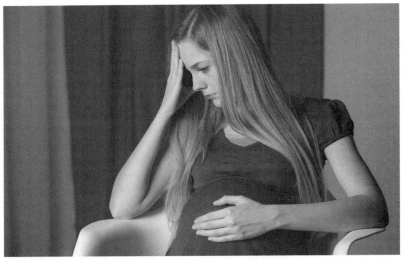

Many are unaware that postpartum depression or anxiety disorders may actually begin *during* pregnancy as well as after a woman has given birth.

cant differences between the two groups of women, most notably, mood changes that were unique to childbirth.

Lack of Resources

Perinatal nurse researcher Dr. Cheryl Beck believes a lack of mental health providers who are informed about the unique psychiatric problems of postpartum disorders is why more obstetric clinicians do not routinely screen for these disorders. Beck explains: "If a mother screens positive for a disorder, then what do the health care professionals do? Not every area has experts in perinatal mood and anxiety disorders."

Childbirth preparation classes often prepare women for the physical complications of delivery—infection and hemorrhage—but many never mention the possibility of postpartum disorders. Yet the complication of a perinatal psychiatric disorder is almost three times greater than the incidence of either of these other two potential physical complications. The rate of postpartum infection after a vaginal delivery is about 3 percent; in contrast, the rate of severe postpartum depression is about 10 to 20 percent among women who have a baby.

Furthermore, our health care system tends to consider our bodies as having either physical problems or mental problems.

This view encourages health care professionals to know only one aspect of health care: physical or mental. When illnesses such as perinatal psychiatric disorders involve both psychological and physical aspects, some of the problems often do not fall within a health care specialist's domain and so the problems often go unrecognized and untreated.

The lack of awareness by health care professionals and the compartmentalization of health care means that, often, those most at risk for developing perinatal psychiatric disorders are not helped. Even though major depressive disorders that occur in the postpartum period are some of the few mental health problems for which we can predict who is most at risk, many women do not receive the treatment they need to prevent more serious problems. Additionally, many women receive treatment only when symptoms get so severe that they are unmanageable. At this stage it takes longer for the symptoms to subside after treatment begins.

Postpartum Disorders Are Not New

Since the time of Hippocrates, we have known that mothers can experience mood changes after delivery. Just as perinatal psychiatric disorders were found in ancient civilizations, they are found worldwide today. Women in both industrialized countries and "undeveloped" countries demonstrate an increased risk of hospitalization for psychiatric reasons after childbirth.

The first medically documented study of emotional disorders after childbirth was conducted in 1838 by a French physician, Dr. Jean-Étienne Dominique Esquirol. Another French physician, Louis Victor Marcé, continued to study these disorders and wrote extensively about them in the mid-1800s. Marcé delineated three kinds of problems related to the postpartum period: problems first seen in pregnancy, those seen immediately after delivery, and those seen about six weeks after delivery. His pioneering work helped clinicians recognize that there is more than one kind of psychiatric problem related to pregnancy and childbirth.

Marcé's work is still viewed today as the first serious attempt to categorize postpartum psychiatric disorders. Marcé also believed that problems in the postpartum period were unique to this time in a woman's life and were distinct from

15

other psychiatric problems outside the postpartum period. The Marcé Society, an international organization devoted to the study and treatment of postpartum disorders, is named in his honor. It is a major source of information and collaboration about postpartum psychiatric disorders worldwide.

In the 1920s, psychiatrists who developed a classification system for psychiatric disorders left out postpartum mood disorders because they did not consider them distinct from other psychiatric disorders. As a result, generations of psychiatric professionals such as psychiatrists, psychiatric nurses, psychologists, and social workers were not fully aware of the psychiatric risks accompanying childbirth.

After Marcé's work, there was little investigation of postpartum psychiatric problems until the 1980s. Then, in the 1990s, the medical community began more research on the topic and developed a subspecialty of psychiatry called *perinatal psychiatry*. Leading medical researchers and clinicians have expanded the knowledge base about the psychiatric problems affecting women during pregnancy and after childbirth. More and more health professionals, as well as the public, are learning about this potentially vulnerable time for a woman's mental health.

2

Postpartum Blues

Maternity blues, baby blues, natal blues, mommy blues, and postpartum blues are all terms used to describe the temporary tearfulness, mood swings, fatigue, and irritability that you might experience in the first few weeks after giving birth. This reaction is common. Paula, a twenty-four-year-old mother, recalls her experience as like being on an emotional roller coaster:

> When I got home from the hospital, I was so happy I was giddy. My baby was perfect. Labor was not as bad as I thought it would be. But, the first day I was home, I burst into tears. I couldn't figure out why I was crying. Then I would be ecstatic. This roller coaster scared me because I could never predict how I was going to feel. I thought I was the only one who ever cried after having a new baby at home. Finally, after ten days, I stopped the crying and began to feel good about myself and the baby.

Symptoms of Postpartum Blues

Many women who have the blues describe themselves as being on a "mood roller coaster." They may feel euphoric and elated, and then their mood plummets to despondency and anxiety. Breaking into tears "for no reason" is common. This frightening, out-of-control feeling adds to their anxiety and fear. Some women understand this pattern of extreme mood swings as a normal reaction to the tremendous physical and psychological changes that go with having a baby. Other women translate the symptoms into a suggestion that they are not good mothers, and they fear they are never going to be good mothers. Many women also worry that their behavior will affect the baby. These unexpected feelings add to the feeling of being out of control.

Postpartum blues usually begin one or two days after delivery and last two to three weeks. Unless they mark the beginning of severe depression, the symptoms of true postpartum blues will subside and you will soon begin to feel more like your old self. However, during these first few weeks, it is difficult to distinguish between depression and the blues. If you have not had a previous depression and if the symptoms are not severe, the health care professionals working with you may want to wait to gauge the severity and longevity of your blues before determining if it is a depressive episode and not the blues.

Causes of Postpartum Blues

Many physical and emotional changes are taking place in your body after your new baby arrives. The cause of the blues is not completely understood, but this time of massive change in your life has some primary "culprits."

Physical Changes

The sheer number of physical changes in your body as you undergo labor and delivery are unparalleled. At no other time in adulthood does the female body experience such a tremendous upheaval. The change in hormone levels from pregnancy to postdelivery is drastic. The stress response to labor and delivery alone can lead to an emotional "letdown." Blood volume, blood pressure, changes in the immune system, and fluctuations in metabolism are just a few of the many changes your body undergoes.

Psychological Changes

The major psychological change that occurs as you adjust to motherhood is also probably unprecedented in your life. Giving birth is a major life event. The abruptness of the change in your life on becoming a parent may be one factor that contributes to maternity blues. Even though the nine-month pregnancy is a preparation of sorts, there is no way to prepare you or your partner for the awesome, yet overwhelming, responsibility of having a child.

Fatigue

Compounding the physical and psychological changes is fatigue. If you had major surgery or had been injured in a car accident, you would be put to bed for rest. But women are expected to have a baby and instantly become an adjusted, loving mother. Because childbirth is a "natural" event, it is perceived that these changes will have little impact on the new mother. Yet the physical and psychological changes of pregnancy and childbirth are in themselves exhausting and overwhelming.

Add to that mix the profound lack of sleep that accompanies having a newborn, and there is sufficient reason why you might feel as if you are on an emotional roller coaster! Nevertheless, fatigue is often understated as a major contributing factor in postpartum blues. Several factors may combine to make you feel overly fatigued: visitors, early discharge from the hospital, lack of support from the extended family, lack of paternity leave for fathers, and the minimization in our culture of the childbirth event itself.

Risk Factors for Postpartum Blues

How to predict who is most at risk for postpartum blues remains unclear. However, the biggest predictor of postpartum blues appears to be a previous episode of the blues. If you have had postpartum blues once, you are at high risk for another episode. The relationship of other mood disorders to postpartum blues is not so clear-cut.

Some professionals believe there is no relationship between postpartum blues and a previous psychiatric illness, such as anxiety, depression, or bipolar disorder. However, Michael O'Hara, Ph.D., past president of the Marcé Society, disagrees. He believes a previous episode of postpartum blues creates an increased risk for another episode. He conducted a study that included women with:

- depression during pregnancy
- at least one previous episode of depression in their lives
- higher levels of premenstrual depression
- a close blood relative with a mood disorder

There may be "technical" reasons why some physicians disagree with Dr. O'Hara's findings. The conflicting views may reflect the lack of a clear definition for the blues and the lack of a consistently valid measurement tool.

If you're having your first baby and you have one or more of these risk factors, realize that you might have the emotional ups and downs of postpartum blues. Also, be sure to discuss any history of past emotional problems or depression with your health care provider.

Tools for Coping with Postpartum Blues

What we tell ourselves about ourselves, our "self-talk," is often something we tend to take rather seriously. Yes, our own opinions of ourselves carry weight. However, when you're not feeling well—as in the case of postpartum blues—it's easy for your thinking and self-talk to become distorted. Accordingly, you might find yourself blaming yourself for dark moods that simply are not the result of you doing anything wrong.

You can use the following tools to take good care of yourself and ignore your negative self-talk.

Don't Blame Yourself

Recognize that *most* women experience the blues to some degree. Your tears, your elation, your fatigue, and your worries are all part of a normal adjustment process to one of the biggest life changes you will ever experience. Paula, a new mother discussed earlier in this chapter, was worried that her blues were a sign that she didn't want to be a mother:

> The experience of having the mood changes was bad enough, but I thought it meant that I had made a big mistake by wanting to be a mother. I thought all mothers who really wanted their babies were happy. Since I wasn't completely happy, I assumed I wasn't meant to be a mother.

It is important not to assign a negative meaning to your symptoms as Paula did. If you assume that you are having these feelings because you are not a good mother, or because you are weak, or because you do not really want a baby, you may actually increase the severity of your symptoms. This can lengthen the time it takes to adjust to your new role as a mother as well as the physical changes your body is undergoing. Instead of listening to such negative "self-talk," remind yourself that your reaction is very typical of that of thousands of new mothers. Perhaps your feelings are signaling that you need to get more rest and pamper yourself a little. If you take care of your emotional and physical needs, your recovery will likely be faster. Our brains often believe what we tell them: tell yours good things.

Get More Rest and Sleep

Getting plenty of rest is the single most important thing you can do to overcome postpartum blues. Many new mothers downplay this advice and say, "Other women don't need this much rest," or "I shouldn't have to spend so much time resting. After all, childbirth is a natural process."

Sleep is required to heal physically, to adjust psychologically, to make milk, and to stabilize your mood. It has been proven that sleep deprivation can drastically alter the mood of healthy people who have not experienced massive physical changes; it can even make people lose touch with reality. Why then, do new mothers assume they are immune to problems that may arise from a lack of sleep?

If you find yourself crying and are not able to identify a reason, don't assume you are doing something wrong. You do not *need* a reason to cry, but you can use the tearfulness and anxiety as a signal that you may likely need more sleep. Everyone has individual sleep needs. Pay attention to yours. Sleep while the baby sleeps. If you need to ask for some help with the baby so you can get more sleep, then do so. To sleep soundly for a few hours, you may even need to get away from the baby. If doing so will help you relax and rest better, make arrangements for someone to take the baby for a stroller ride or a car ride for a few hours. Your baby will benefit from your rest.

If you are having trouble getting enough sleep, perhaps your partner can do the last feeding and put the baby to bed. This will let you get an early start on a good night's sleep. Remember that, even though you are a mother, you are also a person with needs.

Nourish Your Body

In addition to sleep, your other physical needs must be met, including eating well and drinking plenty of liquids. However, this sound advice often goes unheeded. Many women ignore cues from their body about the need for nourishing food.

21

Make You and Your Baby a Priority

The time immediately after childbirth is not the time to tackle home projects like cleaning closets, painting the living room, or doing other things around the house. Joy, a thirty-one-year-old first-time mother, remembers her experience well:

> My friends and family warned me that I was not going to be able to keep the house as clean as I liked after the baby got here, but I didn't believe them. I had always been efficient and kept the house very neat. I was sure I would be able to handle everything. I planned on painting most of the house inside when I was home on maternity leave. As you can imagine, I had to adjust to a new standard of housekeeping, and the house did not get painted!

Allow yourself the first few weeks at home to relax and rest as much as you can, get accustomed to your new routine, and enjoy life with your new baby

Postpone Having Visitors

Tell people who want to visit to wait a few weeks until you and the baby have settled in. If it is hard for you to say no, then use an answering machine to screen calls or allow your helpers to do that for you. If friends and family offer to help, ask them to bring a meal or to come over to dust and vacuum. People like to feel helpful and appreciate concrete suggestions.

If, on the other hand, you need to be in touch with family members and friends, and your friends or relatives are not coming to see you (because they think you want to be left alone), call them! Tell them you are going stir-crazy and ask them to come see you and bring all the latest news.

This is a time to "baby" yourself. Doing so may be difficult because you are so focused on your baby. But remember, your baby needs for you to be healthy and at your best. Our society teaches women to put other people's needs before their own. If this is your pattern, think of a balance between your needs and those of the baby.

Plan an Activity Outside the Home

If you need to get out of the house for a change of scenery, your baby will do just fine in someone else's care for a few hours.

When to Seek Professional Help

If, after a few weeks, your moodiness does not improve or if you are unable to get adequate sleep, then you should seek professional help. However, if at any time you are feeling desperate and fear you cannot continue feeling as you do, call a health care professional immediately. Don't wait a week or two to see if you will start to feel better. At the very least, you will probably experience some relief in talking to a professional about how you feel. And, hopefully, you will also get a professional, objective opinion about what kind of treatment, if any, you may need.

3

Postpartum Depression

Carla, a twenty-six-year-old mother of two, describes a very common experience among new mothers with postpartum depression:

> I had the blues after my first child, but after about three weeks, I got to feeling better. But after my second baby was born, I felt like I never enjoyed her. I resented her crying, and felt like I couldn't get enough sleep.
>
> After two months, I thought I was such a terrible mother that I even wished I were dead. I told my husband how I was feeling. He had noticed I was irritable and had lost a lot of weight. I hadn't realized I was getting so thin.
>
> I called my OB physician, who sent me to a therapist. I was started on medication and went to therapy for a few months. I didn't realize what I was feeling was so serious.

Symptoms of Postpartum Depression

As explained earlier, *postpartum depression* is a term that applies to several psychiatric problems during and after pregnancy. The specific depression in the postpartum period is a mood disorder that affects how we think and feel. Like other kinds of depression, postpartum depression can range from mild to severe. In this chapter, I focus primarily on *major depression*, the most common kind of depression that occurs in the postpartum period. The symptoms must have been present for two weeks to meet the criteria for diagnosis.

Following are some broad categories that characterize symptoms of postpartum depression:

24

Negative Thinking

Thoughts are predominately negative and pessimistic. You may think something like "I can't stand this anymore" or "I will never feel better." Depression can affect our ability to solve problems and think rationally. People who are depressed have problems focusing or expending the effort to concentrate. Sometimes, you might notice that you no longer read the newspaper, or you have stopped reading books.

Depressed Mood

The predominant feelings of depression are hopelessness, sadness, and dejection. Some people describe depression as always being in a gray fog with no bright spots. Others describe it as a "numb" sensation as well as a feeling of not being attached or connected. The pervasive and insidious nature of depression can affect one's judgment, and many people who have depression do not realize how impaired they are.

Physical Symptoms

Depression can affect us physically by altering our sleep patterns, appetite, physical movements, and immune system. Physical aches, such as headaches, may be related to depression. Constant fatigue may also be related to depression. (I know—new mothers are always fatigued!) But constant fatigue even after a good sleep should be questioned.

How Postpartum Depression Is Diagnosed

Diagnosing mood disorders is sometimes difficult because a person may show symptoms of more than one kind of problem. For example, if this is a first-time episode of depressive symptoms, it is hard for the clinician to tell if it is a major depressive episode or a manifestation of the depressive phase of bipolar disorder. And, sometimes, psychotic symptoms are related to a bipolar disorder psychosis, or a brief psychotic episode, and can even be confused with the intrusive thoughts of obsessive-compulsive disorder.

It may take time for the clinician to confirm the exact diagnosis. During this time, various medications may be suggested. This can often be frustrating and confusing for the woman and her family.

Sometimes, clinicians will use a screening tool to help diagnose depression and other mood disorders. The Patient Health Questionnaire-9 (PHQ-9) is a commonly used screening tool to help diagnose depression. This questionnaire is used to monitor the severity of depression and response to treatment.

Patient Health Questionnaire-9 (PHQ-9)

Over the last two weeks, how often have you been bothered by the following problems? (Circle the number to indicate your answer)	Not at all	Several days	More than half the day	Nearly every day
Little interest or pleasure doing things	0	1	2	3
Feeling down, depressed, or hopeless	0	1	2	3
Trouble falling or staying asleep, or sleeping	0	1	2	3
Feeling tired or having little energy	0	1	2	3
Poor appetite or overeating	0	1	2	3
Feeling bad about yourself—or that you are a failure or have let yourself or your family down	0	1	2	3
Trouble concentrating on things, such as reading the newspaper or watching television	0	1	2	3
Moving or speaking so slowly that other people could have noticed? Or the opposite—being so fidgety or restless that you have been moving around a lot more than usual	0	1	2	3
Thoughts that you would be better off dead or of hurting yourself in some way	0	1	2	3

Scoring the Patient Health Questionnaire

After completing the questionnaire, add the total of the numbers you have circled. Depression severity is measured as: 0-4 none, 5-9 mild, 10-14 moderate, 15-19 moderately severe, 20-27 severe. Any positive response to the last question needs to be discussed with a clinician.

Diagnostic Criteria for
Major Depressive Disorder

Most clinicians believe that any depression or anxiety within the first year after delivery is generally associated with postpartum mood disorders.

Mental health clinicians use a standard list of symptoms from *The Diagnostic and Statistical Manual V* to make sure that diagnoses of mental health conditions are consistent across the country. This is a reference book that lists all of the current accepted psychiatric diagnoses and the criteria for each diagnosis. The term *postpartum depression* is not listed as a specific diagnosis in this manual; however, "major depression" is listed.

For a diagnosis of a major depressive disorder to be made, five or more of the following symptoms must have been present during the same two-week period and at least one of the symptoms is either depressed mood or loss of interest or pleasure:

- depressed mood most of the day, nearly every day
- markedly diminished interest or pleasure in all, or almost all activities
- significant change in weight or appetite
- insomnia or hypersomnia (excessive sleepiness)
- (speaking or moving slowly, or the opposite, being fidgety or restless) nearly every day
- fatigue or loss of energy nearly every day
- feelings of worthlessness or excessive or inappropriate guilt nearly every day
- diminished ability to think or concentrate, or indecisiveness
- recurrent thoughts of death, recurrent suicidal thoughts, a suicide attempt, or a specific plan for suicide
- symptoms cause clinically significant distress or impairment in social, occupation, or other important areas of functioning.

The above factors are not attributable to physiological effects of a substance or to another medical condition.

Source: *Diagnostic and Statistical Manual of Mental Disorders.* 2014. 5th Edition. American Psychiatric Association.

How Postpartum Depression Differs
from Other Depressive Disorders

In addition to the previously listed symptoms, there are unique aspects of depression in women who have had a baby.

Negative Perception of Role as a Mother

New mothers with postpartum depression cannot separate their mood problem from their evaluation of themselves as mothers. They have feelings of guilt about being a "bad" mother. They attribute their mood state to not loving their baby enough. These thoughts are the hallmark of postpartum depression and distinguish it from other kinds of depression. Carla describes her experience:

> When I look back at what I was thinking when I was so depressed, it really scares me. The emotional pain was so great that I lost my perspective about me. I never thought I would ever want to kill myself, yet at the time it seemed like such a logical solution to the pain. I still feel guilty that I could ever think about hurting my baby. I still have to work at the idea that those thoughts were depression, not the real me.

One of the most troublesome facets of any kind of depression is that it affects our perception of ourselves and the world. We don't think that something is happening "to" us. Rather, we think we "are" the painful emotions. Carla did not realize she was depressed. She could not objectively observe her negative thoughts and feelings. When you have a cold, you realize there is a change in your health. You say, "I have a cold," rather than "I am a cold." But with depression, you think, "I am depressed," rather than "I have a depression." This perception, as well as the shame and embarrassment often associated with mental illness, often keeps women from talking about their emotional experiences.

Suicidal Thoughts

The most severe form of postpartum depression may bring on suicidal and even homicidal thoughts. When a woman feels so bad that she thinks she cannot take it anymore and that there is no hope for change, the future looks very bleak. When the situation seems hopeless, some women begin to think that they and their baby would be better off dead. This seems like an extreme reaction to those who do not understand the pain and agony of depression. Unfortunately, for anyone who is very depressed, death may seem like a logical alternative.

Causes of Postpartum Depression

Most people find depression difficult to understand. Even more confusing is why the time after having a baby may be so hard for many new mothers. Psychiatric clinicians and researchers are not entirely certain why the postpartum period is a time of high risk for a woman to become depressed, but the following are known to be some of the causes:

Women More Likely than Men to Experience Depression

In general, after adolescence, women are twice as likely to experience depression as men. It is not always possible to determine a single event or problem that may be contributing to a woman's depression. There are many factors—sociological, psychological, and physiological—that contribute to this fact. There may be many reasons. For example, violence, such as rape or sexual abuse, may be a major cause of depression. Women are much more likely to experience such violence than men. Psychological and sociological stress interacts with biology in a way that we do not yet fully understand. You must think of yourself as a whole person, not as a body with a separate mind.

Dana C. Jack, Ed.D., is an internationally known professor and psychologist who is an expert on depression in women. In her book, *Silencing the Self: Women and Depression,* she makes the point: "Depression is a complex and multifaceted illness. By current consensus, major depression results from an interaction of biological and psychosocial factors; no single cause can be isolated."

In other words, Dr. Jack is saying that if you are depressed after giving birth, it does not mean that you are weak or that you are a poor mother. Many factors contribute to how we each experience and react to events.

As mentioned earlier, one of the major predictors for postpartum mood disorders is the prior experience of mood changes during the menstrual cycle. Most research indicates that there may be a hormonal component to some female mood disorders, but our current understanding of the complex hormone system is incomplete. Statistically, the time after childbirth is an adult woman's greatest period of risk for a psychiatric disorder, and it is also the time of greatest fluctuation in hormone levels. Yet, even though all women have similar hormones, not all women experience postpartum mood disorders.

Massive Hormonal Shifts

Abrupt hormonal changes may be a major factor in mood changes after delivery. The complex relationship of your endocrine (hormone) system to moods and thoughts is not yet very well understood, but we do know that during pregnancy, hormone levels are high because the placenta produces hormones. (The *placenta* is an organ attached to the lining of the womb during pregnancy.) Your female hormones—*estrogens* and *progesterones*—are at a very high level.

Your level of male hormones, or *androgens,* is also high because they rise in proportion to the levels of your female hormones. The thyroid gland also increases production of various hormones during pregnancy. At delivery, removal of the placenta and fetus causes a woman's female and male hormone levels to drop drastically. At the same time, *prolactin,* a hormone that promotes milk production, increases. The prolactin level remains high for about two weeks after delivery, regardless of whether you are breastfeeding.

Studies that have evaluated the use of hormones to treat mood changes during the postpartum period are currently inconclusive.

Previous Depression or Anxiety

As we've established, women who have had a previous major depression or anxiety episode are at greater risk of postpartum depression. Why? The "kindling theory" suggests that once a person has a mood disorder, he or she is more susceptible to further episodes of mood disorders. This may be due to a vulnerability to altered levels of chemicals, called *neurotransmitters,* in the brain. This connection is not well understood, and research is ongoing. Carla had an earlier episode of depression in college, although she did not realize its significance at the time:

I remember a time in college when I was depressed for about six months. I barely kept up in class, lost weight, slept a lot, and even lost a lot of my friends. I thought I was just stressed, but now I realize I was de-

pressed. I thought my thoughts of wanting to be dead were just because I was so tired all the time.

Carla's experience is not at all uncommon. Many people can have a mood disorder and not realize what is happening to them.

Genetic Influence

There appears to be a genetic influence on major depression. As yet, the role of genetics and heredity is not well understood. It may be that a genetic vulnerability is why some women are susceptible to the hormonal changes after delivery and other women are not affected. A family history of depression does not automatically mean that you will develop depression or bipolar disorder, but it may mean that you are more susceptible.

Stress and Fatigue

The postpartum period is filled with major stress and fatigue. Whether one or the other causes depression remains unclear. It may very well be an interaction among all the variables.

Stressful events in life, such as moving, job loss, the death of a loved one, or financial reversal, appear to play a significant role in precipitating a depressive episode. Stress may play a role in altering the chemicals in the brain that influence our moods. This phenomenon is not unique to childbearing, but the increased vulnerability and dependency inherent in having a child may place women more at risk.

Relationship Factors

The quality of a woman's relationship with her partner or spouse is another very important variable in determining one's vulnerability to depression. According to several studies, lower levels of marital satisfaction and lack of support are key factors in postpartum depression. If your relationship with your significant other is strained, the new baby in your life may feel like more of a burden or may make you feel more "trapped."

Psychological Adjustment

Psychologically, the postpartum period forces you to assume a new identity and role. Sometimes the baby seems larger than life. You may often feel overwhelmed by the monumental change that has just occurred in your life. Part of this new identity involves adjusting to the changes in your body. All women (in fact, all parents) will have some mixed feelings about this new intrusion and change in their lives. *Ambivalence* may occur even if the pregnancy was very much planned and wanted.

Any change involves loss, and loss includes some conflicting emotions, even when the change is a positive one. Sometimes the baby's arrival even signifies loss. The loss includes the sense of oneself and the loss of the "couple," for now there are three instead of two. Freedom of choice and one's sense of control may be seemingly "stolen" by this new, totally dependent little person. Maybe now you think you will never finish school, get that degree, move to another part of the country, and so on.

The mother's psychological makeup may have some bearing on her tendency to become depressed. Women who have negative, critical, or blaming thoughts about themselves are more likely to become depressed. Women who need to feel in control or to maintain perfectionism are also at risk of depression. Because the postpartum time is particularly stressful, the new mother facing greater responsibilities and lacking typical coping mechanisms will be at risk for postpartum depression.

In his work, *Psychological Aspects of Women's Reproductive Health,* Dr. Michael O'Hara summarizes the various factors that may contribute to postpartum depression:

A composite sketch of the woman who is most likely to be at risk can be developed. The vulnerable pregnant woman is one who has had a past episode of depression (or other serious psychiatric disorder). During pregnancy or after delivery, she may experience some significant negative life events such as loss of housing or loss of employment for herself or her partner. She may be in an unsatisfying relationship with her partner, or she may have no partner to provide support and assistance to her. Finally, during the early postpartum period she may experience the blues, which may persist longer than usual. All of these features will increase the woman's risk for a postpartum depression.

Effects of Mother's Depression on a Baby

The mother-infant connection is vital to the mental and physical health of the baby. Anything that interferes with the critical process of bonding will have a detrimental effect. Depression makes the new mother less able to respond to the needs of the infant.

However, we must not underestimate the hardiness of the baby. Dr. Martin Maldonado, child psychiatrist and professor at the Karl Menninger School of Psychiatry, says, "Babies are quite resilient and don't give up easily. They have a big repertoire of behaviors to make parents respond." He describes several signs that a baby might be affected by a mother's mood changes: mild delays in speech, too placid or content, too irritable, short attention span, feeding difficulties, sleep problems, and a depressed look on the baby's face. "Problems have multiple causes, and it is not helpful to find blame," he cautions parents. Maldonado also proposes that if problems exist for the baby, then attention should be paid to the whole family, especially the mother.

A new mother who is depressed or anxious will not be as sensitive to her baby as a mother who is not depressed. A mother who is depressed will show less affection toward her baby, will be less attentive and responsive to the baby's cues, and may even demonstrate hostile actions toward the baby. *Attunement,* the mother's "knowing" her baby and his or her needs, is crucial in mother-infant relationships. A mother who is depressed or anxious will not be as attuned to the baby. In addition, babies pick up cues from their parents and imitate them. A woman who is depressed will show more negative cues like frowning or not smiling or other unhappy expressions. As a result, the baby will learn a more restricted range of emotional expressions.

It is difficult to predict the impact of the mother's illness on the baby due to the many contributing factors: the severity of her illness, its duration, the number of other people involved with the baby, and the baby's temperament. In general, mothers who are depressed during their baby's first year of life may have a negative impact on their child's development. Various studies have found that the more depressed the mother, the greater the delay in the infant's development. The first year is a particularly critical time for cognitive development. If development is delayed, the effects may still be evident years later.

In the words of Cheryl Beck, Ph.D., a nurse and researcher: "It is imperative that greater attention be paid to a depressed mother and infant. Rapidly developing infants experience the world through those who care for them. Most times, the mother constitutes the primary social environment in the months after birth. Early identification and resolution of postpartum depression will help to alleviate disturbances in mother-infant interactions and enhance the development of warm, sensitive relationships."

Effects of Mother's Depression on Family Members

Postpartum depression involves more people than just the mother and her baby. Other family members will also be confused and concerned. After all, they may think, most women don't feel this way. Relatives may downplay the problem or blame the mother, which can delay treatment. Yet family members are in a unique position to recognize the problem and to help make the new mother aware of her depression. Their lack of knowledge about postpartum mood disorders, however, may prevent them from realizing that this is a real problem that requires treatment to avoid the sometimes tragic consequences.

Sam, a thirty-one-year-old father of two, speaks to the potential tragedy of postpartum mood disorders:

My wife had some problems with crying and thinking she was a bad mother after the birth of our first baby. After our second was born, it was worse. She didn't want to be left alone with the baby and didn't even want to touch it. I had to work, and it was a terrible time for us.

When the baby was one month old, I got a call from my neighbor. My wife had left the kids with her and said she couldn't stand to hurt her kids anymore and left. I didn't see her for about four years, and I didn't know if she was dead or alive. We divorced, and she has very little contact with the children. Later, I found out some information about postpartum depression. I wish I would have known about it earlier. Maybe my kids would have had their mother.

Sam's story is a tragic example of how the lack of information on and treatment for postpartum depression can have devastating results for a family.

Treatment for Postpartum Depression

Once a diagnosis of postpartum depression is made, treatment usually consists of medication, therapy, or a combination of the two. It may not be clear initially which treatment is optimal, but the general consensus is that both together are more effective than either one alone.

If you have never been in therapy or talked with a mental health professional, you will probably feel anxious about this process. The process usually includes an evaluation by a clinician, which involves asking questions about your past medical and psychiatric history, your family history, and the severity and range of your symptoms. The clinician will then determine the diagnosis. Treatment for depression and other disorders will be covered in chapter 8.

The good news is that major depression is a very treatable illness. With prompt treatment, women with postpartum depression tend to improve quickly. In fact, one recent study shows that women with postpartum depression respond faster and require less medication than those with other kinds of depression.

Mood Management Strategies

If you are having problems such as those described in this chapter, the most important step to take is to obtain professional help. There are also several strategies for you to help yourself. However, these are not substitutes for professional guidance.

Become Informed

There is a great deal of information about postpartum depression available on the Internet. Many books are also available both about postpartum disorders and depression in general. In the Resources section of this book there are several Internet sites listed for women coping with postpartum disorders.

Manage Stress

Minimizing stress in your life will help you get better. If you can take an extended leave of absence from work or ask someone to care for your other children for a period of time, you can make your recovery a priority. It is sometimes difficult for mothers to realize that they can help their children and family the most by taking care of themselves first. Although some women seem to handle work and a new baby well, many women need time to adjust and recover.

Ask for Help

Often, women try to hide their symptoms. As a result, family and friends may not realize they are having trouble. Be clear and direct about what you would like people to do for you. Allow others to handle some responsibilities. Give yourself permission to heal. Recovering from a major depressive episode will take longer than you think, and it requires an effort on your part to change. This effort requires energy and concentration that you will not have if you expend your time and energy on chores such as housecleaning and cooking, which other people can do for you.

Eat Nutritious Meals

Eating a healthful diet, avoiding alcohol and caffeine, and getting some physical exercise daily will also help you get better. Now is a good time to incorporate healthful habits into your routine that will not only be physically beneficial but will also help you manage your moods.

Should a Depressed Mother Stop Breastfeeding?

If you are having mood changes and do not feel as well as you think you should, weaning the baby may seem like a solution. In fact, for some women, stopping breastfeeding improves their mood because they are likely to get more rest and may return to a more stable, pre-pregnancy state. Yet, other women notice no difference in their moods upon weaning the baby.

If a woman's mood changes for the worse during weaning, it is likely that she will experience similar problems with weaning after future deliveries. This doesn't mean that weaning is necessarily causing a mood change. The difference in mood may be related to the change in hormones, or it may be a sense of loss that sometimes occurs for women when they stop breastfeeding. Or, the mood change could be due to factors that medical professionals don't yet understand.

Get a Treatment Referral Now

Postpartum Support International (PSI) helps women get help as quickly as possible in all 50 states and in 49 foreign countries. PSI coordinators are trained to answer questions about postpartum depression, to offer telephone support, and to listen for emergency situations. They also will recommend the nearest expert who can diagnose and treat postpartum psychiatric disorders.

To contact PSI, visit their website, www.postpartum. net. Click on "Get Help" and then click on the desired state or country. Or, call the helpline at (800) 944-4773. Someone will answer your call live or return your call within 24 hours.

Consider the story of Paulette, a twenty-eight-year-old mother of two:

I noticed that I became very depressed for about one month after I stopped nursing my first baby. I cried for no reason. I couldn't sleep and generally felt miserable. I thought it was because I missed nursing.

With my second baby, it happened again. I was working then as a nurse. Being an R.N. was a stressful job, and I felt overwhelmed and not able to do my job. When I got very depressed again, to the point where I could not get out of bed or take care of my kids, I knew I needed help.

It is believed that changes in the level of *prolactin*, a hormone present in high levels during breastfeeding, may be responsible for mood changes related to weaning for some women. If you are having problems with your mood, consult a mental health professional before attempting to wean on your own.

Other Mood Disorders

Although major depressive disorder is probably the most common mood disorder during the postpartum period, there are other mood disorders that also cluster at this time.

Dysthymia or Persistent Depressive Disorder

Dysthymia, a persistent depressive mood disorder, is not well known by the general public, but is one of the more common kinds of depression. It is a long-lasting, milder form of depression, but it can have debilitating results. Sometimes, dysthymia becomes worse and increases in severity so that an episode of major depression occurs. Dysthymia is commonly found in people who have suffered trauma such as physical or sexual abuse or neglect in their childhood. Dysthymia can develop during adulthood if stress or trauma such as an abusive relationship continues for a period of time. Many people live with dysthymia for long periods of time, thinking they are just tired or stressed. Sometimes, an inadequately treated major depressive episode will develop into persistent depressive disorder.

Diagnostic Criteria for
Persistent Depressive Disorder

Psychiatrists and psychologists use *The Diagnostic and Statistical Manual V* to diagnose psychiatric disorders, including postpartum disorders. This is a standard set of symptoms that clinicians agree to use to define persistent depressive disorder:

- depressed mood for most of the day, for more days than not, for at least two years
- presence (while depressed) of two or more of the following:
  - poor appetite or overeating
  - insomnia or hypersomnia
  - low energy or fatigue
  - low self-esteem
  - poor concentration or difficulty making decisions
  - feelings of hopelessness
  - There has been a manic (euphoria) or hypomanic (milder euphoria) episode, not attributable to substance abuse or another medical condition.
  - Symptoms cause significant distress or impairment in social, occupational, or other important functions.

Source: *Diagnostic and Statistical Manual of Mental Disorders*. 2014. 5th Edition. American Psychiatric Association.

Bipolar Disorder

Another kind of mood disorder that is similar to major depressive disorder is *bipolar disorder*. Once known as *manic depression,* this disorder is a mental illness that involves vast, out-of-control mood swings from depressed to elevated moods. This extreme high is referred to as *mania* (or a *manic* episode). People who are manic don't realize they are being unreasonable and may do dangerous things. Other symptoms besides mood swings may be not needing to sleep for a period of time, impulsive behaviors such as spending money excessively, and other risky behaviors such as gambling excessively or driving recklessly.

A milder form of this mood state is called *hypomania;* here a person may experience a milder form of mania and then hit a slump and become depressed. People with hypomania realize they are being agitated or unreasonable.

These cycles of bipolar depression may be erratic or regular, and research shows that family history may play a role—a person may have had a family member who has had this illness. It is important for women with severe symptoms to understand this illness because a first diagnosis of bipolar disorder is often made during the postpartum period.

One first-time mother describes the onset of her bipolar disorder:

I guess I have always had mood swings since high school, but they were never serious. Even during pregnancy I would have times of depression and then I would feel fabulous. I even built a chicken coop in our backyard when I was eight months pregnant. After the baby was born, I didn't sleep for four days. I decided to go see the solar eclipse in Nova Scotia, and had booked our plane reservations. I was extremely irritable, and my husband thought it was just from having a baby. Finally a neighbor told him I wasn't acting right and that I should see someone. A psychiatrist diagnosed me with bipolar disorder, and after I was on a mood stabilizer I felt normal for the first time in many years.

Bipolar disorder is uniquely different enough from major depressive disorder that there is a screening tool specific for this fluctuating mood state. It is called the *Mood Disorder Questionnaire (MDQ)* and is commonly used by clinicians in conjunction with another questionnaire, the *Patient Health*

Questionnaire-9 (PHQ-9), (*See* questionnaire on page 26.) to help clarify which mood disorder is present. Remember this is only a screening tool and is not a diagnostic tool.

Diagnosing Bipolar Disorder

There is no single test for diagnosing bipolar disorder. Only in-depth discussions with a clinician can determine whether you might have bipolar depression. Often, clinicians will use the Mood Disorder Questionnaire (MDQ) as a screening tool only.

Mood Disorder Questionnaire

Instructions: Please answer each question to the best of your ability:

1. Has there ever been a period of time when you were not your usual self and...

    you felt so good or so hyper that other people thought you were not your normal self or you were so hyper that you got into trouble?_____Yes_____No

    you were so irritable that you shouted at people or started fights or arguments? _____Yes_____No

    you felt much more self-confident than usual?_____Yes_____No

    you got much less sleep than usual and found you didn't really miss it?_____Yes_____No

    you were much more talkative or spoke much faster than usual? _____Yes_____No

    thoughts raced through your head or you couldn't slow your mind down?_____Yes_____No

    you were so easily distracted by things around you that you had trouble concentrating or staying on track_____Yes_____No

    you had much more energy than usual?_____Yes_____No

    you were much more active or did many more things than usual? _____Yes_____No

    you were much more social or outgoing than usual, for example, you telephoned friends in the middle of the night?_____Yes_____No

    you were much more interested in sex than usual? _____Yes_____No

    you did things that were unusual for you or that other people might have thought were excessive, foolish, or risky?_____Yes_____No

    spending money got you or your family into trouble? _____Yes_____No

40

Mood Disorder Questionnaire (Continued)

2. If you checked YES to more than one of the above, have several of these ever happened during the same period of time? _____ Yes _____ No

3. How much of a problem did any of these cause you—like being unable work; having family, money, or legal troubles; getting into arguments or fights?
____ No Problem ____ Minor Problem ____ Moderate Problem ____ Serious Problem

4. Have any of your blood relatives (i.e. children, siblings, parents, grandparents, aunts, uncles) had manic-depressive illness or bipolar disorder? _____ Yes _____ No

5. Has a health professional ever told you that you have manic-depressive illness or bipolar disorder? _____ Yes _____ No

Sources: The University of Texas Medical Branch. Reprinted by permission. This instrument is designed for screening purposes only and is not to be used as a diagnostic tool.

Scoring the Mood Disorder Questionnaire

There is no specific scoring method for this questionnaire; it is meant to be used to start a discussion between you and your clinician. However, point out to our clinician if you answered "yes" to 7 or more of the first 13 questions. If you answered "yes" to question 2 and "moderate" or "serious" to question 3, be sure to see a clinician for an evaluation.

Diagnostic Criteria
for Bipolar Disorder Diagnosis

The Diagnostic and Statistical Manual V is used to list the symptoms required for the diagnosis of bipolar disorder.

Bipolar I Disorder

Bipolar I disorder is defined by a manic episode alternating with a hypomanic or depressive episode. *Mania* is defined as a distinct period of abnormally and persistently elevated, expansive, or irritable mood and abnormally and persistently increased goal-directed activity. This lasts at least one week and is present most of the day nearly every day. At least one episode of mania is required for the diagnosis of bipolar I disorder.

During the period of mania, three or more of the following are present and represent a noticeable change in behavior:

41

- inflated self-esteem or grandiosity
- decreased need for sleep
- more talkative than usual or a pressure to keep talking
- flight of ideas or racing thoughts
- distractibility
- increase in goal-directed activity (work, school, sexually) or agitation
- excessive involvement in activities that have a high potential for painful consequence, such as unrestrained buying sprees, sexual indiscretions, or foolish business investments

The mood disturbance is sufficiently severe to cause marked impairment in social or occupational functioning. Hospitalization may be necessary. The symptoms are not attributable to the physiological effects of a substance.

Bipolar II
Bipolar II features at least one hypomanic (milder euphoria) episode and a current or past depressive episode.

A hypomanic episode is a distinct period of abnormally and persistently elevated mood lasting at least four consecutive days and present most of the day nearly every day.

During the period of mood disturbance, three or more of the following symptoms have persisted and represent a noticeable change from usual behavior:

- inflated self-esteem or grandiosity
- decreased need for sleep
- more talkative than usual or pressure to keep talking
- flight of ideas or subjective experience that thoughts are racing
- distractibility
- increase in goal-directed activity
- excessive involvement in activities that have a high potential for painful consequences

The episode is associated with a change in functioning that is uncharacteristic and is observable by others.

The episode is usually not severe enough to require hospitalization. The episode is not attributable to the physiological effects of a substance. The condition that accompanies the above criteria is similar to the diagnosis of major depressive disorder.

Source: *Diagnostic and Statistical Manual of Mental Disorders.* 2014. 5th Edition. American Psychiatric Association.

If you are experiencing any of the problems described in this chapter, there is hope. As you can see from the variety of symptoms and diagnoses, the help of a knowledgeable clinician is vital. More treatment options are covered in chapters 7 and 8.

4

Postpartum Anxiety Disorders

Because all new mothers are generally anxious and worried around their new babies, health professionals often overlook more severe anxiety that some women have. There are several types of severe anxiety disorders commonly seen in pregnant and postpartum women.

These anxiety disorders range from the milder *adjustment reaction,* to *generalized anxiety disorder, panic disorder,* and to the more severe *post-traumatic stress disorder.* Before discussing these disorders, let's first examine what I call "normal" anxiety.

"Normal" Anxiety

To understand the various kinds of anxiety disorders that may accompany pregnancy and the postpartum period, it may be helpful for you to first understand the kind of "normal" anxiety that nearly everyone experiences. People with anxiety disorders often report that others minimize or brush off a new mother's problems. This may occur because all people experience anxiety, so they may not understand the difference between anxiety and anxiety disorders.

"Normal" anxiety is a protective response to events outside the range of everyday human experience. It helps us concentrate and focus on tasks. It helps us avoid threatening situations. Anxiety also provides motivation to accomplish things that we may otherwise tend to put off. In fact, anxiety is essential to our survival.

Bodily Reactions to Anxiety

When we are faced with real or imagined threats, our brain signals the body that we are in danger. Hormones are released as part of this general alarm call. These hormones produce the following changes:

- the mind is more alert
- blood-clotting ability increases, preparing for injury
- heart rate increases and blood pressure rises (there may be a sensation of the heart pounding and a tightness in the chest)
- sweating increases to help cool the body
- blood is diverted to the muscles to help prepare for action (this may lead to a light-headed feeling as well as a tingling in the hands)
- digestion slows down (this may lead to a heavy feeling like a "lump" in the stomach, as well as nausea)
- saliva production decreases (which leads to a dry mouth and a choking sensation)
- breathing rate increases (which may feel like shortness of breath)
- liver releases sugar to provide quick energy (which may feel like a "rush")
- sphincter muscles contract to close the opening of the bowel and bladder
- immune response decreases (useful in the short term to let the body respond to a threat, but over time harmful to our health)
- thinking speeds up
- there is a sensation of fear, a desire to move or take action, and an inability to sit still

As suggested by this list of bodily changes, when we have moderate anxiety, our heart rates increase minimally so that there is more oxygen available to our bodies, making us better prepared to take action. We are alert so we can focus better on a task or problem. Our muscles are slightly tensed so we can move and work. Our production of hormones, such as adrenaline and insulin, are slightly elevated to help the body react. We can study for a test, prepare a report for work, give

45

a speech, or hit the ball when we are up to bat. If we were completely relaxed, we could not concentrate or accomplish these tasks as readily. Anxiety helps us meet the demands made on us.

Anxiety is often described as a spectrum of feelings as illustrated in the diagram below. Just about everyone experiences mild or moderate anxiety as we go about our work and play. The feeling we call "anxiety" is accompanied by a predictable pattern of bodily responses summarized in a continuum of anxiety states below.

Ranges of Anxiety

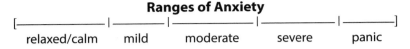

relaxed/calm   mild   moderate   severe   panic

Sometimes, the normal mechanism for initiating these anxiety responses goes awry for reasons we do not fully understand. When we have severe anxiety, we do not think well and cannot solve problems. Production of adrenaline may be so high that it causes a sensation of a "pounding" heart, shortness of breath, and extremely tense muscles. We may feel a sense of danger or dread. This fear may or may not have a focus. If we were facing a tiger, this level of anxiety would be helpful to us to fight or flee. However, if this level of anxiety occurs without a dangerous stimulus, this response is not helpful.

Anxiety Disorders

People with anxiety disorders have anxiety in situations that are not threatening. They experience anxious feelings that are more intense and longer lasting. Anxiety disorders interfere with one's ability to function at work, at play, and in relationships.

All new mothers are somewhat anxious. Being a mother is a new role, with a new person in your life. Anxiety in response to this situation is very common. Pediatricians, obstetricians, and nurses are used to worries, concerns, and questions that new mothers may raise after giving birth.

However, some mothers have excessive worries and experience a severe level of anxiety. Dori, a new mother, describes her anxiety this way:

I could not sit still or relax at all. My thoughts were racing, and I couldn't focus on anything. I worried constantly that something was wrong with the baby or that I would do something wrong. I couldn't even focus to make dinner or finish a load of laundry. I had never felt this kind of anxiety before, but I thought maybe it was normal for new mothers.

As mentioned previously, anxiety disorders often go unnoticed in new mothers because of the common belief that all new mothers are excessively anxious. If you find yourself meeting the criteria for any of the anxiety disorders described in this chapter, or if you are very uncomfortable for prolonged periods, such as for several hours, talk to your health care provider. Take this book with you and share your concerns, because not all health care providers are familiar with the criteria for anxiety disorders. If you have more severe anxiety, particularly for more than a few weeks, you are at increased risk for developing depression and at higher risk for a prolonged illness.

Symptoms of Severe Anxiety

Lack of Joy

As with Dori, mothers with severe anxiety have difficulty enjoying their new babies. They find that, even if it was planned, the new baby is not bringing them enjoyment. This lack of joy often leads to increased self-doubt, and new mothers assume it means they don't love their babies. This can have long-lasting negative effects on their self-esteem and confidence as a mother.

Overly Worried

Women with severe anxiety are overly concerned about minor problems. They have unrealistic fears about doing something to hurt the baby. They are unable to maintain a healthful perspective about what problems are serious and what problems are minor. Mothers with severe anxiety cannot relax even when there is an opportunity to do so.

Mood and Physical Changes

Anxiety and depression are often seen together, and women who are primarily anxious are often also slightly depressed. But sometimes the depression is more severe, especially if the anxiety persists.

47

Anxiety can often lead to sleep interruption, which then can affect energy, concentration, and mood. A problem with sleep is often a common complaint. Sometimes, the gastrointestinal system is affected, causing either constipation or diarrhea. Some women find their milk supply is affected.

Screening for Anxiety

Anxiety disorders are common in the postpartum period. However, many screening tools specific to postpartum do not detect anxiety. Clinicians and researchers in Australia have developed a useful screening tool called the *Perinatal Anxiety Screening Scale (PASS)*. They discovered 80 percent of the women seeking psychiatric treatment had some form of anxiety.

Note that this questionnaire is not a diagnostic tool, but is intended to provide information about the level of anxiety you may be experiencing.

Perinatal Anxiety Screening Scale

☐ANTENATAL (Near time of birth)　　☐POSTNATAL DATE:_____.

Weeks pregnant_____Baby's age_____.

Over the past month, how often have you experienced the following? Please check the response that most closely describes your experience for every question.

	Not at all	Some times	Often	Almost Always
1. Worry about the baby/pregnancy	0	1	2	3
2. Fear that harm will come to the baby	0	1	2	3
3. A sense of dread that something bad is going to happen	0	1	2	3
4. Worry about many things	0	1	2	3
5. Worry about the future	0	1	2	3
6. Feeling overwhelmed	0	1	2	3
7. Really strong fears about things...needles, blood, birth, or pain	0	1	2	3
8. Sudden rushes of extreme fear or discomfort	0	1	2	3
9. Repetitive thoughts that are difficult to stop or control	0	1	2	3

Perinatal Anxiety Screening Scale (Continued)

	Not at all	Some times	Often	Almost Always
10. Difficulty sleeping even when I have the chance to sleep	0	1	2	3
11. Having to do things in a certain way or manner	0	1	2	3
12. Wanting things to be perfect	0	1	2	3
13. Needing to be in control of things	0	1	2	3
14. Difficulty stopping checking or doing things over and over	0	1	2	3
15. Feeling jumpy or easily startled	0	1	2	3
16. Concerns about repeated thoughts	0	1	2	3
17. Being "on guard" or needing to watch out for things	0	1	2	3
18. Upset about repeated memories, dreams, or nightmares	0	1	2	3
19. Worry that I will embarrass myself in front of others	0	1	2	3
20. Fear that others will judge me negatively	0	1	2	3
21. Feeling really uneasy in crowds	0	1	2	3
22. Avoiding social activities because I might be nervous	0	1	2	3
23. Avoiding things can concern me	0	1	2	3
24. Feeling detached like you're watching yourself in a movie	0	1	2	3
25. Losing track of time and can't remember what happened	0	1	2	3
26. Difficulty adjusting to recent changes	0	1	2	3
27. Anxiety getting in the way of being able to do things	0	1	2	3
28. Racing thoughts making it hard to concentrate	0	1	2	3
29. Fear of losing control	0	1	2	3
30. Feeling panicky	0	1	2	3

Perinatal Anxiety Screening Scale (Continued)

	Not at all	Some times	Often	Almost Always
31. Feeling agitated	0	1	2	3
Global Score				

Source: Somerville, S., Dedman, K., Hagan, R., Oxnam, E., Wettinger, M., Byrne, S., Coo, S., Doherty, D., Page, A.C. (2014). The Perinatal Anxiety Screening Scale: development and preliminary validation. Archives of Women's Mental Health, DOI: 10.1007/500737-014-0425-8 © Department of Health, State of Western Australia (2013) Copyright to this material produced by the Western Australian Department of Health belongs to the State of Western Australia, under the provisions of the Copyright Act 1968 (Commonwealth of Australia).

Scoring the Perinatal Anxiety Screening Scale

The Perinatal Anxiety Screening Scale is scored by adding the total of all your responses. The following scores indicate severity of anxiety: asymptomatic (no symptoms of anxiety): 0-20, mild to moderate anxiety: 21-41, severe anxiety: 41-93. A score of 26 or higher may indicate the presence of an anxiety disorder.

Causes of Anxiety Disorders

There is probably no *one* single reason why people develop anxiety disorders. Because we are limited in our understanding of how these disorders develop, it is probably not all that helpful to try to figure out how yours started or whether you inherited these traits. Still, as with depression, there are several theories about why these problems occur.

Biological Predisposition

One theory proposes that some people have a biological tendency toward anxiety. Some people seem to be more sensitive to the effects of the hormones released during pregnancy. There may be a genetic link in some disorders. Because the chemicals in the brain that are affected in anxiety are similar to the ones affected in depression, family history is important in determining what kind of disorder is present and what kind of treatment may help.

Learned Responses

Another theory proposes that anxiety is a learned response to negative or fearful situations as we grow up. If you were around someone who was fearful, negative, and/or critical when you were a child, you may have developed a long-standing habit of assuming the worst is going to happen or you may react negatively to certain events. This theory also explains why trauma, an extremely upsetting event, may play a role in the development of anxiety. If you are in an accident, if you see someone die, or if you are attacked, you may have a reaction that marks the beginning of an anxiety disorder. Reactions to stress and loss may also be a factor.

Physical Factors

If you find yourself fitting the criteria for a diagnosis of an anxiety disorder, it is important that the possible physical causes of these symptoms be eliminated. Several physical illnesses may cause symptoms similar to those of anxiety disorders. A basic principle of mental health treatment is to first rule out any physical causes of symptoms. Some of these physical conditions or illnesses are hypoglycemia (low blood sugar), hyperthyroidism (an overactive thyroid), inner ear problems, mitral valve prolapse (a heart problem), high blood pressure, and some nutritional deficiencies. Although the anxiety symptoms caused by these problems affect only a small percentage of people with the symptoms, it is important to first investigate all the possible physical causes of the symptoms.

Personality Traits

People with anxiety disorders are often known as "worriers" and are overly concerned about control and perfectionism. These can be good traits to have to some extent, but when the need for perfectionism or control interferes with your life, an anxiety disorder often develops.

The following are descriptions of a range of postpartum anxiety disorders.

Adjustment Disorder

Adjustment disorder is a reaction to an external stress beyond what is considered typical. It is usually time-limited and responds well to minimal intervention such as education and psychotherapy. Many people have difficulty accommodating changes in their lives with events such as divorce, job loss, retirement, or other life events. Having a baby is a major change in your life, and you may need time and help to adjust emotionally.

Although it is not specifically an anxiety disorder, adjustment disorder is included in this chapter because anxiety is such a common feature of this condition. However, symptoms of depression may be present also. Twenty-nine-year-old Darla's story is typical of adjustment disorder.

After my son was born, I felt "revved up" and could not sit down and relax for a minute. I felt like there was a motor inside of me that would not shut off. I just thought it was the excitement of having the baby we had wanted for so long. When I got home from the hospital, I couldn't sleep at all. I got so tired and irritable that when the baby cried I wanted to yell, "Shut up!" This only made me feel worse. I was worried I could not handle being a mother. I found myself avoiding taking care of my baby. It took me almost two months before I could enjoy him.

Diagnostic Criteria for
Adjustment Disorder

As with many other psychological problems, adjustment disorder is also diagnosed based on the criteria listed in *The Diagnostic and Statistical Manual V.*

An adjustment disorder is defined as the development of emotional or behavioral symptoms in response to an identifiable stressor occurring within three months of the onset of the stressor. These symptoms or behaviors are clinically significant as evidenced by one or both of the following:

- marked distress that is out of proportion to the severity or intensity of the stressor
- significant impairment in social, occupational, or other important areas of functioning

This stress-related disturbance does not meet the criteria for mental disorder and is not merely a worsening of a preexisting mental disorder.

The symptoms do not represent normal bereavement.

The symptoms do not persist for more than six months.

Source: *Diagnostic and Statistical Manual of Mental Disorders.* 2014. 5th Edition. American Psychiatric Association.

Treatment for Adjustment Disorder

Psychotherapy is typically the preferred treatment for adjustment disorder. Darla, the young mother above, was referred to a therapist who helped her learn to relax and to not worry so much about minor problems such as diaper rash.

Darla tended to "catastrophize." In her thinking, small events took on life-and-death proportions. Darla learned to observe herself catastrophizing and also learned to be more objective in her assessment of situations. After several sessions with the therapist, Darla was less anxious and began to enjoy her baby.

Generalized Anxiety Disorder

A more severe form of anxiety is *generalized anxiety disorder (GAD)*. This illness is characterized by a persistent anxiety that affects most areas of a person's life. This disorder is accompanied by worries or fears that are out of proportion to the situation. Many people, men and women alike, have this kind of anxiety but never seek treatment. They are known to their friends and families as "worriers."

Some women with generalized anxiety disorder may feel less anxiety during pregnancy. For other women, anxiety may continue during pregnancy. It is difficult to predict who will experience anxiety during pregnancy, but if a pregnant woman has had anxiety, she is likely to experience anxiety again after delivery.

Jill's story is typical of a new mother with generalized anxiety disorder:

I have always been a "worry wart" and have been teased about my nervousness since I was a little girl. I felt pretty good during my pregnancy. But after the baby came, I got much worse. I couldn't sleep, and I was always calling the doctor, because I thought something was wrong with the baby. I developed horrible muscle spasms in my neck. The pediatrician suggested I see a therapist about my anxiety. I didn't realize that what I had could be helped.

Diagnostic Criteria for
Generalized Anxiety Disorder

The symptoms of generalized anxiety disorder as listed in *The Diagnostic and Statistical Manual V* are:

Excessive worry and anxiety occurring more days than not for at least six months. The individual finds it difficult to control the worry. The anxiety and worry are associated with three or more of the following six symptoms:

- restlessness or feeling keyed up or on edge
- being easily fatigued
- difficulty concentrating or mind going blank

- irritability
- muscle tension
- sleep disturbance

These symptoms cause clinically significant distress or impairment in social, occupational, or other important areas of functioning.

The disturbance is not attributable to the physiological effects of a substance or another medication condition.

Source: *Diagnostic and Statistical Manual of Mental Disorders*. 2014. 5th Edition. American Psychiatric Association.

When women with these symptoms see a mental health professional, it is common for them to be asked to fill out a variety of screening tools. The primary tool for screening for anxiety is the *Generalized Anxiety Disorder Questionnaire (GAD-7)*. The higher the score, the more severe the anxiety.

GAD-7

Over the last two weeks, how often have you been bothered by the following problems? (Circle the number to indicate your answer)	Not at all	Several days	More than half the day	Nearly every day
Feeling nervous, anxious, or on edge	0	1	2	3
Not being able to stop or control worrying	0	1	2	3
Worrying too much about different things	0	1	2	3
Trouble relaxing	0	1	2	3
Being so restless that it is hard to sit still	0	1	2	3
Becoming easily annoyed or irritable	0	1	2	3
Feeling afraid as if something awful might happen	0	1	2	3

(For office coding: Total Score T_____ = _____ + _____ + _____)

Source: Developed by Drs. Robert L. Spitzer, Janet B.W. Williams, Kurt Kroenke and colleagues, with an educational grant from Pfizer Inc. No permission required to reproduce, translate, display, or distribute.

Scoring the Generalized Anxiety Disorder Questionnaire

Score of: 5 suggests mild anxiety, 10 indicates mild anxiety, and 15 and higher suggests severe anxiety. A score of 10 or greater indicates a need for further evaluation by a professional.

Treatment for Generalized Anxiety Disorder

Jill, the woman just described, meets the criteria for a generalized anxiety disorder. There are two treatment options for this disorder—psychotherapy along with relaxation therapy and medication, but usually both treatments are used together.

Psychotherapy

Jill saw a therapist who used a cognitive therapy approach to help her become more aware of how her thinking increased her anxiety. *Cognitive therapy* is based on the premise that what we think affects our emotions. Jill realized that she tended to think of things as either "black or white, right or wrong." She tended to assume the worst in most situations. Jill also learned to change her habit of negative thinking. After a brief therapy process, Jill was not feeling anxious and was able to enjoy her baby.

Relaxation Therapy

Another tool that therapists use is relaxation therapy. Learning to use relaxation techniques helps promote calmness.

Medication

If Jill had not responded to therapy, or was unable to use relaxation techniques effectively, then medication would have been used. Chapter 8 discusses the use of medications in detail.

Panic Disorder

A more extreme form of anxiety, *panic disorder,* is marked by intense episodes of anxiety, usually accompanied by a fear of impending death. These episodes are called *panic attacks.* After a person has a panic attack, he or she often has an overwhelming fear of future attacks, and will try to prevent them by avoiding many situations that he or she thinks caused the original attack. Panic attacks are a painful and debilitating illness, as illustrated in Melissa's story:

Ten days after I had my son, I had my first experience of thinking I was going to die. I was giving him a bath. Suddenly my heart started pounding. I became dizzy and short of breath. I was so afraid I would pass out that I got on the floor and crawled with the baby into the bedroom. I called my husband, and he came home.

55

I thought I was having a heart attack, so we went to the emergency room. I was crying and worrying about not seeing my baby grow up. They ran tests and told me I had anxiety. I didn't believe them. I called my own doctor, and he ran some more tests.

When I kept having panic attacks, I started reading about panic. I went to a therapist who helped me manage my symptoms and my thinking. Now I can head panic off most of the time. I still can remember how scared I was. It is hard to believe that it was anxiety and that I was not dying. I am still worried about having another attack.

Twenty-eight-year-old Melissa's description of her panic attack is typical of first-time sufferers. Panic attacks are terrifying and are often mistaken for heart attacks or strokes.

Many people have experienced moments of panic in frightening situations such as accidents, but this is a normal response to a situation outside the range of typical human experience. Panic attacks occur even when the situation does not warrant the body responding in such a way.

Causes of Panic Disorder

Sometimes, panic disorder begins "out of the blue," but frequently it can be connected to a stressful event. Often, the panic attack is associated with a certain place or event. For example, let's say you have a panic attack as you're driving and approach a red light. You begin to experience shortness of breath. Your heart may be pounding and thoughts rush through your head such as: What if I pass out? or What if I crash?

In the red light scenario above, the stoplight becomes associated with fear and discomfort. In the future, you will probably begin to avoid stoplights and may take long detours to reach your destination. Avoiding situations that may precipitate a panic attack becomes a way of life that usually becomes more and more restrictive. These avoidance strategies create major problems in a person's life. Many types of situations are seen as dangers to be avoided. The person's world starts becomes smaller and smaller.

Eventually, a person may not be able to leave the house, go into a public building, drive a car, or be around strangers. This creates a fear called *agoraphobia,* which often accompanies panic episodes. Agoraphobia, translated from Greek, means "fear of the marketplace." The condition has been known since the time of the ancient Greeks. Individuals with agoraphobia are usually terrified of leaving their homes alone. They may fear such things as being in public or among crowds, standing in a line, being on a bridge, or traveling in a bus or car. This avoidance of public places severely restricts their lives. Often they will become depressed because they are so isolated. This sense of being alone, terrified, and unable to seek help is a frightening experience.

Kenisha, a twenty-two-year-old new mother, illustrates the emotional devastation that can result from agoraphobia and panic attacks:

> I was driving to the grocery store with the baby for the first time. Six blocks from home, my heart started pounding. I was sweating. I thought I was going to faint. I went back home. I didn't tell anyone because I didn't want to worry them. Somehow I felt ashamed because I thought I should be able to do something as simple as go to the store.
>
> I thought maybe I was still tired from the delivery or was anemic. But it kept happening when I drove, so I made up excuses not to drive. I refused to go out of the house for four months.
>
> Finally my husband got impatient with me and made me go out. We got a sitter and went out. I had a horrible time. I was so scared, I wouldn't let go of my husband's hand.
>
> He made me go to see a counselor, and I found out I was having panic attacks. I never knew other people had the same thing. I was able to control my anxiety by breathing. I only use medication occasionally. But I keep it with me always as sort of a security.

Kenisha's story is all too common. Not only did she have a frightening experience, but she thought she was the only one affected with the problem. Her story also illustrates how people with anxiety may try to hide what is happening to them because they feel a sense of shame. Anxiety becomes a prison that makes their world become smaller and smaller.

Diagnostic Criteria for Panic Disorder

Again, clinicians rely on *The Diagnostic and Statistical Manual V* for the criteria to diagnose panic disorder.

According to the manual, a panic attack is an abrupt surge of intense fear or intense discomfort that reaches a peak within minutes. During this time, four or more of the following symptoms occur:

- palpitations, pounding heart, or accelerated heart rate
- sweating
- trembling or shaking
- sensations of shortness of breath or smothering
- feeling of choking
- chest pain or discomfort
- nausea or abdominal distress
- feeling dizzy, unsteady, light-headed, or faint
- chills or heat sensations
- paresthesia, which is a numbness or tingling sensation
- derealization, which is a feeling of unreality or depersonalization (being detached from oneself)
- fear of losing control or going crazy
- fear of dying

At least one of the attacks has been followed by one month or more of one or both of the following:

- persistent concern or worry about additional panic attacks or their consequences such as losing control or going crazy or having a heart attack
- a significant maladaptive change in behavior related to the attacks

Source: *Diagnostic and Statistical Manual of Mental Disorders.* 2014. 5th Edition. American Psychiatric Association.

Treatment for Panic Disorder

Most people with panic episodes will need professional treatment that will likely consist of medication and psychotherapy. Many people try to control and manage their symptoms on their own, but only make their symptoms worse. If you or someone you know suffers from panic disorder, it is important to seek help immediately. Like depression, panic disorder is very responsive to treatment. Many people have this problem. You are not alone.

Strategies for Managing Panic

In addition to medication and psychotherapy, the following strategies can help lessen and eventually prevent episodes of panic:

Relaxation Breathing Exercise. Most of us use only part of our lung capacity when we breathe. We usually do not use our abdominal muscles. By breathing deep and using your abdominal muscles, you can tell your body and mind, "All is well, and you can relax."

Follow the instructions below to learn this breathing relaxation technique:

- Sit or lie comfortably. Close your eyes or gaze at a fixed spot in the room.

- Begin to focus on your breathing, putting all other thoughts out of your mind. The only thing you have to do now is to practice relaxation breathing.

- Begin to pace your breathing by counting: in...2...3...4 and out... 2...3...4. You can also pace your breathing with positive sayings, such as breathing in and saying, "I am more relaxed and calm." Then repeat it while exhaling.

- Gradually take deeper and deeper breaths, consciously raising your abdomen when you breathe in and lowering your abdomen when you breathe out.

- Continue comfortably breathing for at least ten minutes.

Like any skill, relaxation breathing will take some practice. It is easier to identify the abdominal muscles used for relaxation breathing if you lie on your back with your knees bent and your feet on the floor. Put your hands on your abdomen and concentrate on making your hands rise and fall. The abdomen should rise as you inhale, and fall when you exhale. Try practicing for at least five minutes two or three times daily.

Gradually, you will master this kind of breathing. You can use relaxation breathing to help diminish your anxiety or even to prevent anxiety in situations that might cause you to feel tense. This kind of behavior training is commonly used to help people lessen their reliance on medication.

Progressive Muscle Relaxation Exercise. A similar technique often used in conjunction with relaxation breathing is muscle relaxation. This is usually a guided relaxation exercise; it can be on audio or read to you by someone. You can record the steps yourself, being sure to pace the reading so that you don't rush through it. But you may find it more helpful to have someone read the steps to you slowly, allowing you to concentrate on your breathing and relaxation.

- Sit or lie comfortably. Close your eyes or gaze at a spot in the room. Gradually focus your mind on your breathing.
- Begin to take deeper breaths, raising your abdomen as you breathe in and lowering your abdomen as your breathe out.
- Feel your body relax and become warmer and heavier as you continue the deep breathing. Notice how your body sinks into the chair. Notice your feet touching the floor, and notice your back against the chair. Feel yourself grounded and safe.
- Inhale deeply, curl your toes under on both feet and hold for a count of 1-2-3-4. Relax your toes and take two deep breaths.
- Inhale deeply, curl your toes under again for a count of 1...2...3...4...5...6. Relax and breathe deeply, being sure your abdomen rises as you breathe in and falls as you breathe out.
- Now tighten your calf muscles for a count of 1...2...3...4.
- Relax and take two deep breaths.
- Tighten your calf muscles again for a count of 1...2...3...4...5...6.
- Let go and breathe deeply, making sure your abdomen rises as you breathe in and falls as you breathe out. Continue this tightening-release-tightening-longer-release pattern with your thigh muscles squeezed together, then your buttock muscles, then your abdomen.
- Then continue the pattern by clenching your hands into fists, then bending your forearms to the biceps, then shrugging your shoulders.
- Finish with the facial muscles by squinting your eyes, then opening your mouth as far as possible.

- Be sure to deep-breathe after tensing each muscle group and count in a gentle rhythmic manner, tensing with the second tensing longer than the first.
- Notice how much more relaxed you feel. You feel calm, relaxed, and peaceful. Tell yourself you have just given your body and mind a treat. It feels good.
- Open your eyes when ready.

As with relaxation breathing, consistent practice on a daily basis will develop your capacity to relax in stressful situations.

Post-Traumatic Stress Disorder

The mental health condition known as *post-traumatic stress disorder (PTSD)* is a result of having experienced or observed a terrifying event. Post-traumatic stress disorder was previously thought to be relevant only for soldiers or accident victims, but more recently this disorder has increasingly begun to be recognized as one of the problems women may experience after childbirth. It is estimated that about 5 percent of women who deliver babies may have post-traumatic stress disorder. Also, many women have experienced post-traumatic stress disorder as a result of sexual violence such as rape or childhood sexual abuse.

Causes of Post-Traumatic Stress Disorder

PTSD is a serious and often unrecognized problem for pregnant and postpartum women. The consequences of unrecognized or untreated PTSD include increased possibility of a new mother having anxiety or depression. Impaired maternal-child bonding may also be a risk with post-traumatic stress disorder. The following are several common factors that may contribute to the development of postpartum post-traumatic stress disorder:

Psychiatric Episode. A common cause for PTSD in women is having a psychiatric episode, such as depression, psychosis, or anxiety during pregnancy or after delivery. Although these experiences may not have been life threatening, the woman may experience a loss of control. The associated sense of shame and embarrassment may cause psychiatric problems.

Traumatic or Frightening Event. It is important to understand that trauma during pregnancy may cause post-traumatic stress disorder. The trauma the mother may experience in-

61

cludes such things as not understanding information given to her by her doctor, a difficult or extended pregnancy or labor, unexpected medical procedures needed during the delivery, and potential fetal or infant problems, such as the baby having an increased heart rate.

Health Concerns. A mother's concerns over her own health are also a major risk factor for PTSD. The perception of traumatic or unusual experiences is highly individualistic, and the perspective of the new mother needs to be assessed, not overlooked.

The sense of vulnerability a pregnant woman experiences heightens any potentially negative event during her pregnancy. The process of labor is also a time of vulnerability, and an unexpected course of labor, such as an unplanned C-section or even an unexpected amount of pain, can cause a stress reaction.

Sarita's story is fairly typical of unrecognized post-traumatic stress disorder:

> This was my third and probably last pregnancy. Both of my two previous pregnancies were very normal. During the tenth week, we had what was described as typical genetic screening. We hadn't done this before. We were told the results indicated the baby might have a severe genetic disorder and that we should consider aborting. More tests were run, and then I was told I had gestational diabetes. I couldn't sleep, and I thought I was going to lose my mind. The next results came back with the baby being okay, but I had to watch my diet for the rest of the pregnancy.
>
> Still, I spent the next few months worrying every minute. When the baby came and she was fine, I couldn't really feel anything for her. I didn't want to take care of her or breastfeed like I did with my two previous babies.

Sarita was given the Edinburgh Postnatal Depression Screening Scale and her score indicated mild depression. It wasn't until she was talking to one of the nurses at her baby's twelve-week checkup that the staff realized she may have post-traumatic stress disorder. The Edinburgh Scale doesn't ask about nightmares. Sarita continued:

> I didn't feel depressed, but I felt numb. Every night I was having nightmares about the baby dying and about me dying. I wasn't sleeping,

and I dreaded going to sleep. I kept having images of the doctor telling me that my baby had a genetic defect.

Diagnostic Criteria for
Post-Traumatic Stress Disorder

As with previous anxiety disorders discussed, the symptoms listed in *The Diagnostic and Statistical Manual V* are used to help clarify a diagnosis of post-traumatic stress disorder. In addition, it is important to ask a new mother questions such as the following about her symptoms as well as about the experience that may have caused the symptoms:

- recurrent, involuntary, and intrusive distressing memories of the traumatic event

- recurrent distressing dreams related to the traumatic event

- flashbacks, which are dissociative reactions in which the person feels or acts as if the traumatic event was happening again

- psychological distress upon exposure to cues that are related to the traumatic event

- physiological reactions to cues that are related to the traumatic event

- persistent avoidance of stimuli related to the traumatic event

- negative alterations in cognition and mood associated with the traumatic event

- marked alteration in arousal and reactivity associated with the traumatic events, such as irritability, outbursts, hypervigilance, sleep disturbance, problems with concentration, and exaggerated startle response

Source: *Diagnostic and Statistical Manual of Mental Disorders.* 2014. 5th Edition. American Psychiatric Association.

Treatment for Post-Traumatic Stress Disorder

A wide variety of treatments are available for those suffering with post-traumatic stress disorder. These treatments consist of group and individual therapy that is tailored for the individual. Many times, medication can be helpful, particularly if sleep is disturbed.

5

Postpartum Psychosis

As discussed earlier, postpartum depression refers to a range of mood disorders. On one end of the spectrum, we have the "baby blues," which usually involves a milder fluctuation in mood for only a short time—maybe one or two weeks. However, at the other end of the spectrum is postpartum psychosis, the most severe form of postpartum disorders.

Postpartum psychosis is a psychiatric emergency. If the psychosis goes unrecognized and untreated, the mother may harm her baby or herself. About 5 percent of women who have postpartum psychosis will kill themselves. This tragedy can often be prevented by obstetric and pediatric clinicians recognizing the signs of postpartum psychosis and treating the new mother. Most instances of postpartum psychosis occur in the first two weeks after the baby is born, with about half of these developing within the first three days.

What Is Postpartum Psychosis?

Postpartum psychosis is a form of mental illness in which a new mother may experience delusions, hallucinations, confusion, and disorganized thoughts or behaviors. *Delusions* are ideas that are false, such as the notion that someone has bugged your house and is listening to you or that your baby has been possessed by an evil spirit. *Hallucinations* usually involve seeing or hearing things that are not there and sometimes feeling things that are not real. Examples of hallucinations are seeing faces in the wallpaper, or hearing a voice telling you to stab your baby. Postpartum psychosis is an uncommon but severe illness that can have devastating consequences for the new mother and her infant. A psychotic episode can be frightening for both the mother and the family; the sense of shame and embarrassment about such irrational behavior can leave a lasting legacy in a family.

However, women who have postpartum psychosis typically recover faster than women who have psychotic episodes at other times in their lives. Still, after such an event, it can be difficult for family members to regain trust in the new mother, even if she is totally recovered. For many years later, any erratic behavior may be viewed with suspicion by family and friends.

How Common Is Postpartum Psychosis?

This disorder occurs in about 1 to 2 women per 1,000 who give birth. (That is less than 1 percent.) Who's at risk? Women who have relatives with bipolar disorder or a psychotic disorder, or have a family member with a previous episode of psychosis in the postpartum period.

Symptoms of Postpartum Psychosis

Postpartum psychosis has a wide variation of symptoms, and not all psychotic episodes are the same. The onset of postpartum psychosis is typically earlier than postpartum depression. Symptoms usually emerge within three to ten days after delivery. Early symptoms include: extreme restlessness, agitation, insomnia, hallucinations, and delusions; a new mother may complain of being confused, disoriented, or "feeling strange." For some women, after giving birth is the first time they have psychotic symptoms and for some it is the first time they have any psychiatric condition at all.

The following story from June, a registered nurse in an obstetrician's office, describes one of her clinic's patients who was having postpartum psychosis:

> We got a call from the husband of one of our patients, who came home from a business trip and found his wife putting their four-day-old baby in the trash bin. The baby was filthy and hungry and had been neglected. His wife was claiming the baby had been taken by Satan. The mother was psychotic. She was dirty, confused, and had a raging breast infection.
>
> We hospitalized her. She responded very quickly and was home within a week. She was mortified at what she had done. We really had to

work with her to let her know that she was ill and that we knew she loved her baby. The sad thing is, her sister had a similar problem, but she never told our patient, so she did not know about this illness.

Diagnosing Postpartum Psychosis

One difficulty in detecting a psychotic state is that there may be periods when a woman is more in touch with reality. In addition, sometimes, women do not reveal that they are having strange thoughts and experiences.

It might be helpful to look at it this way: when psychosis appears, it is a symptom—much like fever. Your doctor may not be sure what is causing the fever, and treats the symptom as he or she determines the causes. It's the same with postpartum psychosis. A woman will be treated for psychosis, and it may be that the cause is a previously undiagnosed or undeveloped bipolar disorder, extreme sleep deprivation, depression, or maybe the mother has an electrolyte disturbance (electrolytes are chemicals in the blood that regulate heart and neurological function, fluid balance, and oxygen delivery). Or perhaps a new mother is having a brief psychotic episode that does not appear to be related to any previous life experiences and will never happen again.

Diagnostic Criteria for Postpartum Psychosis

As with other depressive disorders, *The Diagnostic and Statistical Manual V* is used to define the symptoms that are agreed upon for diagnosing postpartum psychosis:

- delusions
- hallucinations
- disorganized speech
- grossly disorganized behavior

The symptoms last at least one day and less than one month and are not related to a bipolar disorder diagnosis. The psychosis begins within the first four days after a woman's baby is born, but any psychotic episode that occurs after this is also considered to be a postpartum psychosis. A psychotic episode is a symptom of mental illness characterized by radical changes in personality, impaired functioning, and a distorted or nonexistent sense of reality.

Source: *Diagnostic and Statistical Manual of Mental Disorders.* 2014. 5th Edition. American Psychiatric Association.

Another new mother, Sonya, remembers her experience with postpartum psychosis:

> I don't remember much, except that I was agitated, both physically and mentally. My thoughts were racing, and I could not focus on any one thing. I even remember some thoughts I had about the baby being evil, and I thought I saw yellow vapor come from his mouth. I did not know anything was wrong, and no one else realized it for several days after I was home. I look back now and am terrified about what could have happened.

A woman who is becoming psychotic will begin to behave in a noticeably bizarre manner. Both the baby and the mother are at risk during this time because the new mother's judgment is quite impaired. This illness should be considered an emergency, and urgent measures must be taken to bring the situation under control.

Avoiding Tragedy

In June of 2014, *The New York Times* newspaper published a series of articles on the range of psychiatric problems seen in women after delivery. In one of the articles the writer described a woman who was a highly regarded professional in her field. After the birth of her first baby she "became obsessed with the idea that she had caused him irrevocable brain damage." There was no foundation to this belief, but no physician could convince her otherwise. This is a symptom of psychosis called a *delusion*. This woman felt so bad about causing her son brain damage that when he was ten months old she strapped him to her chest and she jumped out of an eighth-floor window in her New York apartment. The woman died, but her son was cushioned from the fall and survived.

Knowledge of the potential danger that psychosis brings to both the woman and baby is sorely lacking in the medical community. Several states have mandates that women be screened for postpartum disorders and that professionals be educated about the associated psychiatric disorders.

Treatment for Postpartum Psychosis

After a correct diagnosis, most women respond rapidly to treatment and can quickly resume care of their children. Treatment will usually involve medication, likely an antipsychotic and perhaps a mood stabilizer. (*See* chapter 8.) Sleep is essential so medication to help a mother sleep will probably be a part of the plan. If symptoms don't diminish quickly, sometimes *electroconvulsive therapy (ECT)* is used. This is a procedure in which electrical currents are administered to the brain. With some mental illnesses, the electronic currents seem to create changes in brain chemistry, resulting is a rather quick elimination of symptoms. The procedure is performed under general anesthesia because it produces a seizure in the person undergoing the treatment.

Still, postpartum psychosis presents a crisis for the family. The aftereffects of postpartum psychosis may last much longer than the psychosis itself. As explained earlier, once a new mother has had a psychotic episode, both she and her family typically may remain anxious for years, fearing that the illness will suddenly return.

Sonya, expressed her ongoing concern this way:

> It took me a long time to get over the shame of having postpartum psychosis. I kept watching myself for signs that I might not be over it. I never want to go through that again, but I want to have another baby. We haven't decided what to do.

The husband and other relatives may not understand what is happening if this is the woman's first episode of psychiatric difficulties. Most families think that the illness indicates the mother will never be able to care for her baby, which is not true. Sonya's husband, Guy, describes his fears:

> I thought I had lost my wife and would have to raise the baby myself. I had never heard of postpartum psychosis, so I thought she would always be hallucinating and delusional. I was so relieved when she became her old self again. But I will never forget how scared I was that Sonya would never get any better.

Risks of Future Postpartum Psychosis

Most women will never have another episode of psychosis unless they have another baby. Then their risk of a second episode of postpartum psychosis is significant. If a woman is at risk for postpartum psychotic episodes, all of her health care providers should be so informed. For those women who have had a psychotic episode, the risk of a subsequent episode is about 50 percent, according to medical researchers. One study shows the risk to be 100 percent if the previous episode occurred within the past twenty-four months.

Prevention of Postpartum Psychosis

There have been some attempts to prevent recurrences in women known to be at risk for postpartum psychosis. But these preventive measures have been based on small groups of women, so further research is needed. Dr. Deborah Sichel was one of the first researchers to report on the use of estrogen after delivery to prevent the development of mood disorders. She suggests that the change in estrogen levels after delivery may cause an "estrogen withdrawal state" that causes the extreme mood swings and psychosis.

Because Dr. Sichel's study involved a small number of women, however, caution is advised in using estrogen after delivery until more research is completed. Although more recent studies also discuss the use of hormones as a preventive measure, the evidence is still not strong enough to make this a standard treatment.

Another approach is to start treatment with medications (mood stabilizers or atypical antipsychotics) immediately after delivery. The mother should also be under very close supervision.

Research is ongoing for this troubling illness that makes the time after the birth of a baby much different from what parents expected. It is important to not assume that the new mother who has a psychotic episode is "forever changed" or is not fit to be a mother. And for women who have had this illness, accepting that a physiological change precipitated this psychiatric illness will be essential for future self-esteem and self-confidence. This event is traumatizing for the whole family, and health professionals must be aware of the potential impact of the illness long after the symptoms are gone.

6

Obsessive-Compulsive Disorder

The psychiatric disorder known as *obsessive-compulsive disorder (OCD)* is often the brunt of jokes about people who are organized, punctual, and perhaps rigid in their habits. But this disorder, which is much more than these characteristics, can have devastating effects on people. The development of obsessive-compulsive symptoms in pregnant or postpartum women is great enough to warrant an examination of this illness. There seem to be specific kinds of obsessions and compulsions in the time before and after the birth of a baby, but it is not clear if this is a distinct type of illness from women with OCD who are not pregnant.

Collette's experience with OCD is all too common:

Collette was an assistant principal at a high school, and she loved her work. She was considered to be the "go-to" person to get things done. She was known for her organizational skills and her attention to detail. Collette planned her pregnancy so that she could deliver after school was out for the summer; she wanted to be able to spend a lot of time with the baby. There were times when Collette felt overwhelmed with trying to keep up with her job and get ready for a new baby, but everyone assured her that her feeling overwhelmed was quite typical. The pregnancy went well, and she delivered on schedule.

About three weeks after delivery, Collette's mother left, after having spent ten days helping out. One evening, Collette was fixing dinner and watching the baby when she was startled by the thought: I'm going to stab the baby. She glanced at the knife on the counter and then fled from the kitchen.

She locked herself and her baby in the upstairs bathroom where she sat down and cried. Her husband found her there when he got home from work. He reassured her she would never do such a thing, and Collette and the baby went back downstairs. Collette was fearful of the knife, so her husband finished preparing the evening meal.

The next day, Collette was so uncomfortable around knives that she put every knife from the kitchen in the trunk of her car, locked the trunk, and put the keys in the basement. She was able to prepare meals using a plastic knife. Her husband became impatient but went along with her. Collette then had difficulty going to her best friend's house with the baby because her friend had a knife block full of knives on the kitchen counter. Collette also had symptoms of moderate depression, exacerbated by not being able to sleep.

Collette came to me for treatment; she was deeply ashamed of having had thoughts of hurting her baby. She thought it meant she was a terrible mother. When I explained the symptom was really a part of her overconscientious mothering, she was greatly relieved.

Many women with OCD are like Collette—they hide their symptoms and are afraid to tell others, which make the symptoms more intense. Collette was a high-achieving, successful woman who had never been diagnosed with a psychiatric disorder previously. But in looking back, Collette recognized that she had always had a need for order and perfection, and when she did not feel in control of her environment, she would become more anxious. Collette's compulsive organizing of her home and office and her extensive list making was an adaptive mechanism—behaviors developed over time—that helped her be successful.

But when she became overwhelmed with adjusting to having a new baby and the physiological changes she was undergoing, her level of OCD worsened. Her thoughts were a result of her creative imagination when it came to thinking of "what harm may happen to her baby." She obsessed about the possibilities. Collette required medication and psychotherapy.

Most women are conscientious mothers, but some can become excessively conscientious. They anticipate danger, and their fear of danger may be so powerful that their perception of reality becomes blurred.

Diagnostic Criteria for
Obsessive-Compulsive Disorder

There are two components to OCD: thoughts or obsessions, and behaviors, which are compulsions—actions we feel "driven" to do. *The Diagnostic and Statistical Manual V* lists the following criteria for diagnosis:

Obsessions are defined by:

- recurrent and persistent thoughts, impulses, or images that are experienced as intrusive and inappropriate and cause anxiety or distress

- thoughts, impulses, or images that are not simply excessive worries about real-life problems

- attempts to ignore or suppress such thoughts, impulses, or images

- awareness that the obsessional thoughts, impulses, or images are a product of his or her own mind

Compulsions are defined by:

- repetitive behaviors (hand-washing, ordering, checking) or mental acts (praying, counting, repeating words silently) that the person feels driven to perform in response to an obsession, or according to rules that must be applied rigidly

- behaviors or mental acts aimed at preventing or reducing distress or preventing some dreaded event or situation

- The obsessions or compulsions are time-consuming, or cause clinically significant distress or impairment in social, occupational, or other important areas of functioning.

- The obsessive-compulsive symptoms are not attributable to the physiological effects of a substance or another medical condition.

In order to meet the criteria for a diagnosis of obsessive-compulsive disorder, either compulsions or obsessions can be present. In addition, at some point, a person with OCD has recognized that the obsessions or compulsions are excessive or unreasonable. The obsessions or compulsions cause marked distress, are time-consuming, and may significantly interfere with the person's normal routine, occupational functions, social activities, and relationships.

Source: *Diagnostic and Statistical Manual of Mental Disorders.* 2014. 5th Edition. American Psychiatric Association.

Characteristics of Postpartum OCD

Some researchers believe that OCD is more common for women in the postpartum period than in comparable groups of women who are not postpartum. It is not clear why this is such a vulnerable time for women. Postpartum OCD has several unique characteristics.

Fear of Hurting the Baby

Many women are like Collette and have intrusive thoughts of hurting their babies. Knives are a frequent trigger, but so are plastic bags, sharp corners, and even water—for fear of drowning the baby. Because OCD is not a psychotic illness, the mother is aware of her actions and is unlikely to act on her thoughts, so there is generally little risk to the infant.

Similarly, some women may obsess about previously having killed a baby; these are often women who may have terminated an earlier pregnancy or have miscarried.

Shame and Secrecy

The new mother often thinks she is the only one who has ever had these intrusive thoughts, and she feels deeply ashamed. A new mother going through this tries mightily to suppress and ignore her thoughts. She may take avoidance measures, such as taking the baby and going to a mall, a library, or a coffee shop. Being away from the home may help her avoid any thoughts of hurting the baby. Some women feign being ill as a way to avoid taking care of the baby; they'll ask someone to come in to care for the infant.

The emotional toll OCD takes on a mother is profound. Many women never forget the thoughts that were so troublesome. Some women with children who are now adults clearly remember the thoughts they had of possibly harming their babies. They still feel the shame and guilt decades later.

Compulsive Behaviors

Sometimes, a woman will become obsessed with cleaning and orderliness. For example, she may compulsively clean and sanitize every counter surface in her home in order to avoid having the baby come into contact with germs. These compulsive actions are strategies to suppress thoughts of harming the baby, and the obsession may interfere with actually caring for the baby. Other types of obsessions that are common are an excessive need for order and symmetry which can also become emotionally debilitating.

Worsening of Mild OCD

Sometimes, women who develop postpartum OCD have had the illness for much of their lives but because it was mild, they were able to keep it hidden. Nola, a twenty-five-year-old mother, tells her story about being afraid she would hurt her infant:

> After I was home for about two weeks, I began having fears about smothering the baby with her pillow. I could not stop the thoughts from happening. I love my daughter so much, and I felt so ashamed of having these awful thoughts.
>
> Finally, I called a crisis hotline. They told me I probably had OCD, and that it was fairly common and treatable. They referred me to a psychiatrist. I was started on a medication, and the thoughts stopped. It was such a relief!

Nola's story is very typical of people with OCD. They recognize that their thinking and behavior is "not normal." As Nola goes on to describe, she—like many women—hid her ritualist behaviors and obsessive thoughts from her family and friends:

> I'd had obsessions since I was a child, but thought I could control them. I never told anyone because I was afraid they would send me to a psychiatric hospital. I used to have to count to a certain number before I opened a door. People would look at me when I hesitated before opening doors. And I also had some compulsions about how things in my bedroom and in the bathroom had to be arranged. At one time, I compulsively used sanitizer on my hands, but had to stop when I developed a terrible infection. I realize now how much of my life I have spent hiding something that was easily treated. I wish I had gotten help sooner so that I would not have had such a hard time when my daughter was born.

Like Nola, many women suffer in silence because they feel so ashamed of having such thoughts

OCD May Occur with Other Disorders

OCD is also highly *comorbid,* meaning it is very common that OCD is accompanied by or is a part of another disorder, such as depression, bipolar disorder, or anxiety disorders. This makes OCD more difficult to treat. Treatment options are based on the symptom profile, so when a woman has a combination of disorders, there is no "one-size-fits-all" treatment with medication and psychotherapy.

It's known that there is a relationship between OCD and bipolar disorder in a significant percent of people. A careful history and close monitoring of postpartum women is important because the first line of treatment for OCD is often an antidepressant, and, sometimes, women who also have bipolar disorder get worse because the antidepressant destabilizes their mood. Consequently, other drugs—mood stabilizers, used to treat bipolar disorder—are often helpful to women with OCD.

The Difference between OCD and Psychosis

It is important to examine the difference between OCD and postpartum psychosis (which is discussed in detail in chapter 5). Women with OCD have some understanding and insight about the origin of their thoughts. They may still consider their thoughts of harming the baby "bizarre" and "frightening," but they understand that they are having the thoughts, and know to not act on the thoughts.

However, women who have postpartum psychosis may have thoughts of harming their babies, but they don't understand the difference between their thoughts and their actions. As a result, they may actually harm the baby. Clinicians need to be able to distinguish between these two disorders. Early in the development of the medical understanding of postpartum disorders, thoughts of harming the baby were thought to be part of a psychotic process. We now know that many more women have OCD than psychosis. As explained in chapter 5, postpartum psychosis is an emergency and must be treated immediately to keep both the baby and the mother safe.

Treatment for Obsessive-Compulsive Disorder

Most women with OCD with likely require medication. Antidepressants, the same medications to treat depression and anxiety disorders, work for OCD as well. Sometimes, the woman will also receive psychotherapy. OCD can take a while to improve, but with diligence and persistence an effective treatment plan can be administered.

7
Psychotherapy
for Postpartum Disorders

I knew I needed help. I had read several books about depression when I was trying to figure out why I was crying all the time, couldn't get things done, and didn't want to be around my baby. My sister had some depression once, and she went to a therapist. But I had no idea how to find someone that I could trust. I called my doctor, and he gave me some names. I was really scared because I didn't know what to expect. I was also afraid of the stigma of "mental illness."

Amanda, new mother

Amanda's lack of knowledge about mental health professionals and her apprehension about getting help for her depression are common experiences among women suffering from postpartum depression or anxiety. Seeking treatment can be unsettling when you are not familiar with psychiatric professionals and your options for care. This chapter is your guide to psychiatric treatment. Actually, many of the ways health professionals treat postpartum disorders are similar to the standard treatments for depression and anxiety in others who are not new mothers.

Meeting with a Mental Health Professional
Whether you are referred to a specific mental health professional or you are calling an agency on your own, you can expect to encounter a similar process.

You will be asked to come in the clinician's office to register, which is similar to the kind of paperwork required by obstetricians and other health care providers. You will need to provide a photo identification and insurance papers.

Psychotherapy for Postpartum Disorders

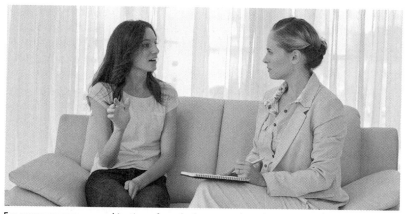

For many woman, a combination of psychotherapy and medication can hasten the recovery process. Choose a therapist who has experience in counseling women with postpartum depression and anxiety.

Your Evaluation

You will meet with an "intake" professional, who may be the mental health professional with whom you will work. During this intake or consultation session, you will be asked a series of in-depth questions. The intake session will usually last forty-five to sixty minutes so that the mental health professional will have enough time to understand not only your current symptoms but also how those symptoms compare with how you felt at earlier times in your life. Another reason for in-depth questioning is that psychiatric symptoms can have multiple causes, so it is important for the professional to understand as much about you as possible.

During a counseling session, common intake interview questions include:

- Why are you seeking treatment?
- What are your current symptoms?
- What is your past psychiatric history?
- What is your past medical history?
- What medications are you are taking? Do you have drug allergies, and past illnesses or surgeries? Use of caffeine, alcohol, nicotine, and other substances, including herbs and supplements?

- What is your family history? The clinician may prepare a *genogram,* a type of family tree. Questions will focus on past and present relationships in your family, any history of drug abuse, family use of alcohol and drugs, and psychiatric and medical illnesses.
- What is your current life like? Your work, social activities, interests, support systems, relationships, and any stresses in your life?

Questions will also focus on your memory and thought patterns.

Getting a Diagnosis

A thorough medical history will be taken because it is standard practice in psychiatric treatment to rule out any physical causes. Many medical disorders, including hypothyroidism, hyperthyroidism, and anemia, can cause symptoms of depression and anxiety. Laboratory or blood tests may also be recommended. After obtaining your history and current concerns, a mental health clinician will then likely make a diagnosis as well as suggest options for treatment. To determine the diagnosis, the mental health professional will consult *The Diagnostic and Statistical Manual V,* used by mental health professionals to ensure consistency in diagnosis. Most insurance companies require the diagnoses listed in this manual for payment.

If you do not agree with or are concerned about either the diagnosis or the recommendations, then you should seek a second opinion. The decision about any recommended psychiatric treatment is yours to make.

Developing a Treatment Plan

After the diagnosis is reached, your mental health care professional will recommend a treatment plan. Sometimes it is as simple as scheduling you for psychotherapy sessions and perhaps starting you on a medication. There are advantages to combining therapy and medication in the treatment of depression or anxiety. Psychotherapy will help relieve your mood disorder, and it also teaches you to recognize the risk factors and indicators of future mood disorders. Medications, such as antidepressants or mood stabilizers, may help you be more responsive to therapy. (Medications will be discussed at length in chapter 8.) A mental health professional is knowledgeable about the wide range of treatment options.

Types of Mental Health Professionals

There are five main groups of mental health professionals from whom you might commonly seek treatment for a postpartum disorder: psychiatrists, advanced practice nurses, social workers, and psychologists. All five of the primary types of mental health professionals are licensed by the state in which they live or practice, so the titles and requirements among states vary. Each professional group has a national certifying body that assures minimum standards. Certification is generally not required to practice, however.

Make sure you understand the credentials of mental health professionals so you can make an informed decision about the right therapist for you.

Psychiatrist

A *psychiatrist* is a physician who has completed medical school and has a medical degree (M.D.). A psychiatrist may also have doctor of osteopathy (D.O.) degree. Both types of doctors must complete a *residency,* which typically takes four years. Both types must also pass the same exams before they are licensed to treat people and prescribe medications.

Be sure the psychiatrist you consult has completed a residency in psychiatry. Psychiatrists may be nationally certified.

Advanced Practice Nurse

A second type of mental health professional is an *advanced practice nurse;* these are registered nurses with a master's degree in psychiatric nursing. Graduate preparation includes a clinical internship in a mental health setting. (An *internship* is a period in one's training in which he or she spends time observing other professionals as they treat patients; another part of an internship involves direct contact with patients.)

These nurses may also be called *clinical nurse specialists* or *advanced registered nurse practitioners.* They can prescribe medications for common psychiatric disorders. These nurses usually have a certification if their state recognizes advanced practice nurses. There is a voluntary national certification program for child and adolescent advanced practice nurses and for adult advanced practice nurses. Some nurses may also have a Ph.D. or a doctorate of nursing practice (D.N.P.).

Social Worker

A *social worker* is a master's degree–level graduate who has completed a clinical internship as part of a graduate program. Some social workers are not clinically trained but instead provide other kinds of services. Other titles in this category include *licensed specialist clinical social worker (LSCSW)* and *clinical social worker (CSW)*. There is a voluntary national certification for social workers. Some social workers may also have a Ph.D.

Mental Health Counselor

These counselors are usually master degree–level therapists. Their education and licensing requirements vary by state. These counselors often work with consulting professionals who will prescribe medication.

Psychologist

A *psychologist* may have a doctorate in clinical psychology. These professionals must have completed a graduate academic program with a clinical component. Those with doctoral degrees may be referred to as having a Ph.D. or Psy.D.

Some states recognize master's-degree programs in psychology. These graduates are also known as psychologists. Be sure either the master's or Ph.D–level clinician you consult has clinical graduate program experience. There is national certification for psychologists.

Other Professionals

Other professionals also may offer therapy; these include marriage/family therapists, ministers, and licensed counselors. Their qualifications may vary. In some states psychotherapy is unregulated, so anyone may call him- or herself a *psychotherapist* (but not a *psychologist*).

Which Type of Mental Health Professional Should I See?

Deciding on a mental health professional can be difficult. Unlike the medical field, where roles are more distinct, many kinds of mental health clinicians do much the same kind of work. According to *Consumer Reports,* 4,000 readers responded to a survey on satisfaction with mental health providers. The results stated: "People were just as satisfied and reported similar progress whether they saw a social worker, psychologist, or a psychiatrist."

Your choice of therapists may depend on the availability of clinicians in your area. Another factor is the cost of treatment. If you are paying for treatment yourself, master's-level clinicians such as advanced practice nurses and social workers may be less expensive. If you have insurance, your policy may dictate which kind of professional you can see. Two types of providers can prescribe medication: psychiatrists and advanced practice nurses. It is not uncommon for a person to see both a clinician who cannot prescribe (such as a social worker or psychologist) for therapy and a clinician who prescribes medication.

To further add to the confusion in this field, there are several different kinds of theoretical approaches that may be used by the five primary mental health providers. In fact, many clinicians use a combination of approaches, describing themselves as *eclectic,* meaning they draw from various schools of thought in treating patients.

What to Look for in a Mental Health Professional

When consulting a mental health professional, you are like any other consumer in search of and paying for a service. You should ask questions, check credentials, and obtain references. You should also interview more than one professional, because it may not be easy to determine who is best for you. Only you can determine if you trust and feel comfortable with someone. It is generally not a good idea to go to a professional you know personally or have business contact with.

One resource for finding mental health professionals is Postpartum Support International, a support organization which is listed in the Resources section in the back of the book. This organization provides therapy referrals as well as information about postpartum problems. They may have information about someone in your area who is knowledgeable about treating postpartum disorders.

After you have met with a mental health professional, ask yourself these questions:

- Did I feel comfortable talking with him or her? Was I able to be completely open?

- Did I feel that I was being judged or criticized?
- Was the therapist able to help me understand my problem and the plan for treatment, or am I just as confused as before we met?
- Was the focus on me or on the therapist?

You will be better able to answer these questions after consulting more than one mental health professional.

Common Approaches to Psychotherapy for Postpartum Disorders

Two common therapy approaches are most often used for depression and anxiety: *cognitive-behavioral therapy* and *interpersonal therapy*. There are other, less common, approaches. *Group therapy* is often used in additional to individual therapy.

How do you decide which approach is best? Unfortunately, no research has shown exactly which therapies are best for certain problems. This is very much an individual decision. One factor to consider is your history. If this is the first time you have experienced symptoms of depression or anxiety, and you do not have a history of trauma (such as neglect, physical abuse, or sexual abuse), then a shorter period of therapy may be the best course of action.

Relieving the symptoms of your current problem should be the first goal of your treatment. Initial treatment should not focus on your conflicts with your mother or your ambivalence about having a baby. If the initial treatment does not help you feel better, then you can look at the historical factors that may be affecting you.

If anxiety is the primary symptom, many clinicians recommend a cognitive-behavioral approach as the treatment of choice. Because most clinicians use a variety of approaches, be sure to ask which approach the professional is going to use and what the rationale is for that choice.

After you have found a mental health professional who is helpful and trustworthy, you may be prescribed medication. A variety of medications are available to treat postpartum disorders. *See* chapter 8 for a discussion of various medications.

Cognitive-Behavioral Therapy

Cognitive-behavioral therapy is based on the premise that how we feel is based on how we think. So, the focus of therapy is on examining thoughts and beliefs and "reframing" them so that we learn to adopt behaviors that are healthier for us. The relationship of thoughts, feelings, and behaviors on the belief system formed by early childhood experiences will be a primary focus. The basic premise is that depression and anxiety are the result of faulty conclusions formed during childhood. Change can occur by learning new responses and new habits.

Cognitive-behavioral therapy's focus is on changing behaviors that are unhealthy for you. The therapist views therapy as a collaborative process and interacts with the patient, providing feedback. Homework assignments may be given to facilitate change.

Interpersonal Therapy

Interpersonal therapy is based on a trusting relationship between you and the therapist. The basic premise is that there is a connection between your mood disorder and the current interpersonal relationships in your life. Change occurs by correcting dysfunctional behaviors within a therapeutic relationship. The therapist will be supportive, warm, and understanding, and will focus much of the work on the interaction between the two of you. This kind of therapy may take longer because it takes a while for trust and a relationship to develop.

Group Therapy

Group therapy is another treatment option and involves several patients meeting with one or more therapists in a group setting. The groups may be time-limited or ongoing. They may be structured, meaning there is a set format or agenda for each group session, or the group may be unstructured, which means that the therapist is not directive but will provide some guidance for the group. Group therapy is usually cost-effective, so managed-care companies encourage participation. Group therapy has the advantage of decreasing the sense of isolation that accompanies depression and anxiety. It has the disadvantage of less individual time that is tailored specifically to your own needs.

Group therapy alone is probably not the best treatment for you initially if you meet the criteria for depression or anxiety disorders. However, it may be a very useful addition to your individual therapy.

Effectiveness of Group Therapy. Few studies have examined the effects of group treatment on postpartum depression. In one prominent study, however, ten group therapy participants were observed over a ten-week period. The group format involved education, social support, and cognitive-behavioral therapy. When self-esteem testing scores of women in the treatment group were compared with the those of women who received no treatment, the group therapy participants scored significantly higher.

If you decide to try group therapy, be sure to first ask about the purpose of the group. If the group is designed to educate, support, and promote change toward healthful behaviors, then it may be helpful. But if the purpose is not clearly stated and the time frame is open-ended, you may want to instead choose a type of treatment more immediately helpful to you.

A Final Note about Psychotherapies

Whatever therapy you decide is best for you, there are some commonalities that make sense for all types of therapy. According to mental health professionals Ivan Miller, Ph.D., and Gabor Keitner, M.D., the therapy should:

- be clear about the rationale for treatment
- establish a time limit, probably weekly sessions for twelve to twenty-four weeks
- employ a therapist who is active and directive
- focus on current problems
- emphasize changing current behavior
- teach self-monitoring of change
- include homework assignments to facilitate application of what is learned to daily life problems

If this is your first time seeking psychiatric treatment, the process can be overwhelming. But, one thing should be paramount: The person helping you should be educating and encouraging.

8

Treatment:
Medication and Non-Medication

If you are suffering with a postpartum disorder, the good news is that a variety of medications are available that can give you relatively quick relief from some emotionally painful symptoms. The severity and longevity of your symptoms are the factors in determining whether you would benefit from medication.

If you have experienced anxiety or depression over a period of several weeks or months, taking medication may be wise. If your symptoms are so severe that you are having trouble taking care of yourself or your baby, or if you are having suicidal thoughts, medication is recommended.

Reluctance to Take Psychiatric Medications

Several factors cause many women to be concerned about using medications while they are pregnant or breastfeeding. First and foremost on the minds of these women is the question: Is it safe for my baby if I take psychiatric drugs? Other issues include a woman's lack of understanding about how the drugs work, believing they need to "try harder" to recover without drugs, and fear of addiction.

Safety Concerns

Are medications safe during pregnancy and breastfeeding? Unfortunately, there is no simple answer. It depends on the medication, how far along you are in your pregnancy, and whether you're breastfeeding. This decision requires a discussion with your health care professional about the risks and the benefits of taking medication. Women who are depressed

85

How Many Women Take Drugs During Pregnancy?

It's estimated that as many as 10 percent of women in the United States take drugs for depression while they are pregnant. The percentage likely rises for postpartum women who have delivered their babies.

---

while pregnant need to realize that their mood disorder may impact their babies as much or more than medication could. Postpartum mothers who are depressed or anxious may not realize the impact their untreated illness is having on their child. Babies born to women who are clinically depressed are more likely to be premature, have lower birth rates, and may be at risk for developmental delays.

Like many women with postpartum depression, Amanda gained some benefit from psychotherapy, but she also required medication to fully treat her symptoms:

> I found a good therapist who helped me feel less depressed, but she recommended that I take an antidepressant in addition to coming to therapy. I didn't want to take medication—I was afraid I might get sicker. My therapist gave me some reading material, and I finally understood how the medication works. I saw a psychiatrist who explained why I needed medications. I am glad I agreed to take the medication. It helped me feel so much better.

As a psychotherapist, I often encounter women in severe distress who say, "I need help, but I don't want to take medication." I usually agree to try therapy first, but if they are not feeling significantly better after two or three sessions, I usually recommend medication. Note that research about medications to treat mental disorders is ongoing, and new medications are always coming on the market. Although some medications have been used successfully, others should be avoided by pregnant and postpartum women. Rely on your prescribing clinician for the most current and most appropriate choice for you.

Lack of Understanding

Many women don't understand how medications for depression work. They view psychiatric medication very differently from other medications. Yet these same women willingly take antibiotics or over-the-counter medications. I believe their

---

**Pregnant Women's Concerns
about Taking Psychiatric Drugs**

- Concern for the baby's safety
- Mother's difficulty weighing her own health against that of the baby
- A lack of information about medications
- Negative external influences, such as a partner who does not want the woman to take medication
- Emotional upheaval in deciding whether to take medications at a stressful time

Source: Department of Psychiatry, Women's College Research Institute, and University Health of Toronto University

---

fear of psychiatric medication is based on a lack of information or even on misinformation.

A note of caution: the Internet is a wonderful resource that is full of information, but you'll also find inaccurate information on many websites, so be selective about which sites you visit. The Resources section at the end of this book recommends reliable websites.

False Belief That They Need to "Try Harder"

Another reason some women don't want to take medication for psychiatric problems is that they view their illness as a weakness. Many people with depression or anxiety tell me, "I should be able to fix this myself without having to rely on medication."

I then ask them, "If you had diabetes or anemia, would you expect to fix it yourself? If you have an infection, do you expect to overcome the infection by willpower?" I then explain the changes in the brain related to depression or anxiety (*see* text on brain chemistry later in this chapter).

Fear of Addiction

Yet another reason some people fear taking psychiatric drugs is their fear of becoming addicted to them. However, because psychiatric medications help restore your brain chemistry to its normal state, you would not become addicted to these drugs. However, drugs that can become addictive include narcotics for pain and some medications used for anxiety, so use of these medications should be carefully monitored by your health care provider.

Brain Chemistry
When You're Depressed or Anxious

Although the brain is still a mystery to us in many ways, we know more today than ever before how our brain chemistry affects our thoughts and feelings. The brain is composed of more than 100 billion nerve cells called *neurons*. These nerve cells transmit information through electrical and chemical functions. Every thought, action, and feeling is the result of these functions throughout the brain. Depression and anxiety are thought to be the results of an excess of, or deficiency in, either the chemical activity or the electrical activity of the brain.

Most of what we call "mental illness" is an alteration in the neurological or chemical functioning of the brain. The psychiatric disorders discussed in this book are really "brain disorders." Researchers have created depression in laboratory animals by exposing them to prolonged stress, such as noise, temperature changes, and flashing lights. After a period of time, the animals resemble humans who are depressed. They lose interest in playing, they don't move about in their cages, they won't eat, and they won't greet the attendants as they used to. Prolonged stress does cause physical changes in the brain and in the body.

Role of Neurotransmitters

Neurotransmitters are the chemical messengers of the brain. Although there are more than fifty known kinds of neurotransmitters, for the purposes of understanding what happens when we are depressed and anxious, let's focus on the primary neurotransmitters that affect mood and anxiety: *dopamine, norepinephrine, serotonin,* and transmitters of *GABA* and *glutamate.* These neurotransmitters work together to regulate our thinking, emotions, and behaviors.

Dopamine is important in learning, memory, and emotional arousal. You probably have had a frightening experience in your life that you remember vividly. Dopamine is involved in helping you remember the event in detail. In fact, you might even be able to remember smells, sounds, or other sensory information associated with the experience. Without dopamine, you would not be able to remember events in such detail.

Norepinephrine is very similar to *adrenaline,* the hormone released during stress. Lack of this chemical may be related to

Medication Effects on Nerve Cells

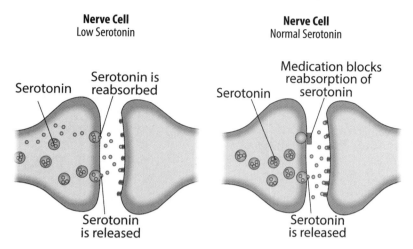

Nerve Cell
Low Serotonin

Serotonin — Serotonin is reabsorbed

Serotonin is released

Nerve Cell
Normal Serotonin

Serotonin — Medication blocks reabsorption of serotonin

Serotonin is released

The low serotonin level, shown between nerve cells above, is associated with depression.

The normal level of serotonin between cells is associated with improved mood. Note how the medication blocks the serotonin from being reabsorbed.

depression. Too much of this same chemical may be related to a state of agitation or mania.

Serotonin seems to play a role in influencing how excited our brain cells get and in helping us fall asleep. Serotonin also plays a major role in regulating mood.

GABA resembles serotonin in that it helps regulate how fast the messages are sent along the nerve cells. Its role is very important because anxiety is considered to be a process of excessive stimulation. A related neurotransmitter, *glutamate,* performs the opposite action. Medications that affect the levels of these neurotransmitters will enhance or inhibit brain activity.

In addition to these major neurotransmitters, *endorphins* play a role in regulating mood. These small proteins seem to promote a sense of well-being and happiness. Exercise increases the production and release of endorphins.

Changes in Hormones

As mentioned previously, the functioning of the thyroid gland may be a factor in postpartum depression. For some reason, massive changes in the body's chemistry can affect the functions of the entire endocrine system, including the thyroid. Hormones—both the female estrogen and progesterone and the male hormone testosterone—seem to influence the normal function of nerve cells and can affect mood; however, the role of the endocrine system in mood regulation is not yet fully understood. In addition, a stress hormone such as *cortisol* may play a major role in the development of depression and anxiety.

Thyroid disorders are often overlooked as a factor in postpartum mood changes. If your health care provider has not ordered a lab test to evaluate your thyroid function, be sure to ask about it.

How Psychiatric Medications Work

Medications target cells in the brain that affect mood, anxiety, and behavior. Antidepressants, for example, increase the amount of the neurotransmitters, such as serotonin, available in the synapses—the spaces between nerve cells in the brain. Whenever symptoms of depression or anxiety appear, there is usually too much or too little of one or more of the neurotransmitters.

The diagram of nerve cells on page 89 shows how the chemicals in a medication affect the receptor sites on brain cells. Even though there is an immediate increase in the level of neurotransmitters in the brain, it sometimes takes weeks before there is a change in mood or anxiety. So the effect on the receptor site is only the first step in a cascade of changes in the brain that will hopefully relieve symptoms.

Many women who are taking antidepressants decide to stop them once they discover they are pregnant, which often can be several weeks past the date of conception. Depending on the medication, stopping the medication is generally not recommended. I tell these women, "The horse is out of the barn." The fetus has already been exposed to the drug during the very early stage of the pregnancy, and the risk of relapse for the mother is too great.

Unless there is a compelling reason to discontinue the medication, with a few exceptions, continuation of the medication is unlikely to cause harm to the fetus. If the decision is made to discontinue the medication, tapering off the drug slowly is best to avoid recurrent symptoms of depression.

Which Medication Is Best for Me?

Your nurse practitioner or physician will ask you questions about your general health, medications you're currently taking, and those you've taken in the past. They may require a blood test and other diagnostic/screening tests. The medications used to treat anxiety and depression are distributed throughout the body, not just the brain. For this reason, it is essential that you report which other medications you are taking. Because some medications do not mix well, possible interactions must be considered.

Knowing which psychiatric medication will work for you is not clear cut. For example, some antidepressants work well if a major symptom is tearfulness. A different antidepressant will probably be used when a major symptom is insomnia. Sometimes it is difficult to know which medication will work for you and which one you can tolerate best.

A trial-and-error approach can be frustrating, but this method often helps in finding the medications that work best for you. Your prescriber will "target" certain symptoms, and will monitor you for changes in your symptoms. You may also be prescribed various dosages since medications vary in strength. For example, you might take 100 milligrams of one medication but need a dose of 250 milligrams of another medication. This dose variance does not mean that one medication is stronger or better. It is just that their chemical compositions differ. The dose determined for each medication is based on how it affects your body.

Medication Side Effects

Side effects must be considered when determining whether to take any drug. All medications carry some risk of side effects, and this concerns some individuals. For example, aspirin is irritating to the stomachs of some people even as it helps alleviate headache or reduce fever. Some antibiotics have side effects that make them difficult to take.

When deciding whether to take a drug, the benefit must outweigh the risks, including side effects. When you are being given a recommendation for a medication, ask about both po-

91

tential benefits as well as potential side effects. But just because a side effect is listed doesn't mean you will have it.

Most antidepressants have side effects, but they will usually diminish. For example, some of them may cause a feeling of "jitteriness" at first; however, this feeling will usually disappear after a few days. If you are having side effects, don't stop a medication until you talk with your health care professional.

Your prescribing clinician will discuss the side effects that you are likely to experience. Side effects with antidepressants, for example, are usually temporary and should go away as your body adjusts to them. Your prescriber should also tell you about any serious or lasting side effects that would require immediate medical attention.

Understand Any Drugs You're Taking

When your physician is explaining a drug he or she is prescribing, take notes about the drug or ask for written information about each drug. During an office visit, it can be difficult to remember all the information a clinician may give you about a drug and its side effects. Your clinician may give you a symptom rating sheet to help you monitor your symptoms and any side effects. It is extremely important that you not change the dose or stop taking the medication without talking first to your prescribing clinician.

If you are seeing other health care professionals for other health problems, be sure to tell each of your physicians about all of your medications. If you use over-the-counter medications or supplements, ask your pharmacist about potential drug interactions before taking them.

Commonly Prescribed Antidepressants

One of the most popular classes of antidepressants are called *selective serotonin reuptake inhibitors,* or *SSRIs.* These drugs prevent the reabsorption, or reuptake, of serotonin in the brain. In other words, the drugs increase the serotonin levels in your brain.

These are the drugs most often prescribed for depression and anxiety; they are the first choice of clinicians for two reasons. First, they have fewer side effects than some of the older antidepressants. Second, laboratory testing is not required before you can take them.

Selective Serotonin Reuptake Inhibitors (SSRIs)
- paroxetine *(Paxil)*
- fluoxetine *(Prozac)*
- fluvoxamine *(Luvox)*
- sertraline *(Zoloft)*
- citalopram *(Celexa)*
- escitalopram *(Lexapro)*

Side Effects of SSRIs. Common side effects from SSRIs include:
- difficulty falling asleep
- feeling "jittery"
- problems with sexual functioning
- upset stomach
- dizziness
- tremors
- lack of sexual desire

Note that most of these side effects are temporary—they go away after a short period of time. One possible exception is a lack of sexual desire and the inability to achieve orgasm, especially if the medication dosage is high. If the side effects do not lessen, the medication may not be the right one for you.

Other medications may be given to counteract the side effects so that you do not have to stop taking a medication that is effective for your depression. It cannot be overstated: it is be dangerous to stop an antidepressant abruptly because doing so may cause sudden changes in your brain chemistry, causing you to feel much worse.

Preliminary evidence in one study shows that women suffering a first-time episode of depression in the postpartum period may respond more quickly and better to SSRIs. The same study also reports that women who started treatment within four weeks postpartum responded more quickly to the medication than did women who started treatment more than four weeks postpartum.

SSRIs' Effect on Babies. There is some preliminary data that SSRI antidepressants use in pregnancy could have a positive effect on the infant, especially in anxious mothers. Infants of mothers who were anxious and took medication were more ready to interact with a toy than were a group of babies born to mothers who did not take antidepressants during pregnancy.

In Canada, an encouraging study did a comprehensive review of seven different studies involving 1,774 women. The researchers found that women taking drugs for depression during pregnancy had no more risk for having a baby with birth defects than women who weren't taking antidepressants.

Other Common Antidepressants

There are several other kinds of antidepressants available. The following list includes medications that are commonly used for depression. These medications target neurotransmitters either in addition to serotonin or instead of serotonin. These drugs listed below may be added to your antidepressant by your prescribing clinician. Some of them are more sedating and can be helpful if you are having a problem sleeping.

- venlafaxine *(Effexor* and *Effexor XR)*
- mirtazapine *(Remeron)*
- nefazadone (no brand available in the U.S.)
- bupropion *(Wellbutrin, Wellbutrin SR,* and *Wellbutrin XL)*
- duloxetine *(Cymbalta)*
- vilazodone *(Viibryd)*
- levomilnacipran *(Fetzima)*
- vortioxetine *(Trintellix)*

Side Effects

The side effects of the antidepressants above are varied because they target a variety of neurotransmitters or have different mechanisms of action in the brain. Talk to your prescribing clinician about possible side effects of these medications.

Tricyclic Antidepressants

The class of drugs known as *tricyclic antidepressants* are "older" medications, used when SSRIs and other medications listed above are not effective; or sometimes, they are used in addition to SSRIs. The tricyclics are effective, but their side effects make them less tolerable for some. These medications require an *electrocardiogram (EKG)* to evaluate heart function if you are over age forty or have a history of heart problems.

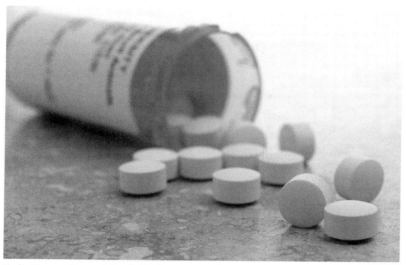

Medications can be a useful and effective treatment for perinatal psychiatric disorders.

Also, it commonly takes four to six weeks before these drugs start to take effect. Of the several medications in this category, the most commonly used ones are listed below.

- amitriptyline *(Elavil)*
- desipramine *(Norpramin)*
- nortriptyline *(Pamelor)*

Side Effects of Tricyclics

The most common side effects of tricyclic antidepressants are a dry mouth and constipation. These can usually be treated by increasing your fluid intake or using a stool softener. Additional side effects include dizziness, changes in sex drive, problems urinating, and weight gain.

Commonly Prescribed Antianxiety Drugs

Several medications, including some antidepressants such as SSRIs, may help treat both anxiety and depression. Sometimes, people whose main symptom is anxiety are surprised to be prescribed an antidepressant, but antidepressants' effect on serotonin levels generally helps anxiety. One of the most common medications used specifically for anxiety is benzodiazepines.

95

Benzodiazepines

Benzodiazepines are tranquilizers prescribed for panic and severe anxiety. They are very popular because they are effective and relatively inexpensive. They work quickly and provide symptom relief immediately, while some antidepressants takes weeks to become effective.

There are short-acting benzodiazepines and longer-acting benzodiazepines. The effects of short-acting benzodiazepine generally last a few hours, although for some people it can last longer. The effects of long-acting benzodiazepine can last six to ten hours. The most commonly used benzodiazepine are:

Short-acting Benzodiazepines

- alprazolam *(Xanax)*
- clonazepam *(Klonopin)*
- lorazepam *(Ativan)*

Longer-acting Benzodiazepines

- diazepam *(Valium)*

Tolerance and Risk of Addiction

A disadvantage of benzodiazepines is that you may develop a tolerance to them and will require higher and higher doses. *Tolerance* means that the original dosage that worked for you initially will no longer be as effective as time goes by, and you'll feel the need to increase the dose. The more frequently you take the medication, the sooner you will develop tolerance. Therefore, these drugs potentially are very addictive. They are to be used with caution and preferably only on a short-term basis.

If you have a history of drug abuse, including the use of alcohol, marijuana, nicotine, or other substances, be sure to let your health care provider know. A past history of addiction does not mean that you absolutely cannot take benzodiazepines. It just means that they must be used with caution.

Some people avoid benzodiazepines. Used carefully, however, they can be very helpful in managing the symptoms of panic and severe anxiety.

Benzodiazepines: Take Only When Needed

An advantage of benzodiazepines is that you can use them as needed rather than take them routinely every day. For some people, a regular dose one or more times a day is recommended at the beginning of treatment. As symptoms subside or as you gain skill in managing your anxiety, you can sometimes start taking these medications only when you feel anxious. It is very important not to abruptly discontinue these medications if you have been taking a daily dose.

Side Effects of Benzodiazepines

The primary side effects you might notice when you start taking benzodiazepines are sleepiness, light-headedness, and sometimes unsteadiness. Do not drive or operate machines until you know how you respond to these drugs. These side effects should become less noticeable as you continue to take these medications. If side effects do continue, talk to your prescriber about reducing your dosage.

It is also important to talk with your prescriber before stopping a benzodiazepine. He or she may wish to gradually taper you off the medication, depending on how long you've been taking it.

Other Antianxiety Drugs

Buspirone

Buspirone *(BuSpar)* is another drug used to treat anxiety. Technically it is a *nonbenzodiazepine;* it affects different brain cells and has no potential for addiction.

Side effects include dizziness, headaches, drowsiness, and nausea. You may have to take Buspirone for a few weeks before it begins to alleviate anxiety. There is little data available about using this medication while pregnant or breastfeeding.

Vistaril

Vistaril or (hydroxyzine) is another medication used to treat anxiety and may be useful especially when the risk of addiction or tolerance is high with benzodiazepines.

The most common side effects are drowsiness and dry mouth.

Commonly Prescribed Mood Stabilizers

For some women, the mood disorder that manifests during pregnancy or postpartum is called *bipolar disorder* or *manic-depressive illness.* This illness requires a medication that will even out your mood and will prevent the "highs," or ma-

97

nia, that accompany mood swings. These medications are also sometimes used to help your antidepressant work better even if you haven't been diagnosed with bipolar disorder. More than one medication may be used to help stabilize mood. The following are commonly prescribed mood stabilizers:

- lithium carbonate *(Eskalith, Lithobid, Lithonate)*
- divalproex sodium *(Depakote, Depakote ER)*
- valproic acid *(Depakene)*
- lamotrigine *(Lamictal, Lamictal XR)*

With the exception of lamotrigine, these medications require that you undergo laboratory tests before taking the first dose to determine if you can safely take them. Without such testing and ongoing monitoring, it is possible for dosages to shift from therapeutic to toxic levels, causing damage to internal organs.

Side Effects of Mood Stabilizers
These medications are generally well tolerated. In higher dosages, they may cause drowsiness.

Atypical Antipsychotics
One of the biggest changes in medications over the past twenty years is the use of *atypical antipsychotic* medications. These medications should really be called "multimodal" medications. They are used for much more than treating psychosis.

These medications are used (in addition to antidepressants) as mood stabilizers and for anxiety management. They are also used for psychotic symptoms during and after pregnancy. However, because these medications are relatively new, their use in pregnant and postpartum women has not been studied extensively.

The following are atypical antipsychotics:

- aripiprazole *(Abilify)*
- asenapine *(Saphris)*
- lurasidone *(Latuda)*
- olanzapine *(Zyprexa)*
- quetiapine *(Seroquel)*
- risperidone *(Risperdal)*
- ziprasidone *(Geodon)*

A national pregnancy registry was established when clinicians started prescribing these drugs. (*See* the reference in the Resources section at the end of this book.) In one study, more than a thousand women who used antipsychotic medications in the first or second trimester were compared with a thousand women who did not use these medications. The study found that these antipsychotics did not increase "short-term" problems for the baby. Nor did it cause problems for the mother such as gestational diabetes, high blood pressure in pregnancy, or blood-clotting problems.

Further, the rate of premature births or infant birth weights did not differ between the two groups of women. This study was done on a group of women in Canada who used publicly funded health care; these women are typically at more risk for health issues because of socioeconomic and health status.

Although we know of the relative short-term safety of these medications, we still do not know the long-term risks. The risks and benefits must be weighed before they should be prescribed. Most clinicians will not use these medications as first options for postpartum depression.

Side Effects of Atypical Antipsychotics

As a class, atypical antipsychotics have a risk of a permanent movement disorder called *tardive dyskinesia,* especially if used long term and at higher doses. The risk is much less than with the older class of antipsychotics, which are not frequently prescribed anymore but are still available and used occasionally. Also, some of these medications have a propensity to cause weight gain and require laboratory work to monitor the effects of the medication on blood sugar and lipids.

What If I Am Breastfeeding?

Breastfeeding is recommended for many reasons by many groups, such as the American Academy of Pediatrics and the American Congress of Obstetricians and Gynecologists. Many medications can be safely used while the new mother is lactating. Most medications will end up in small amounts in the breast milk, and there are guidelines for using medications during lactation. Discuss these with your mental health professional. You may be advised to watch your baby carefully for any signs he or she may be affected by the medication you are taking.

Keep in mind that the infant will be affected by your depression and your anxiety. So, again, in deciding whether to take medications while breastfeeding your baby, discuss the risks and benefits with your prescribing clinician.

Some women who want to minimize exposing their infant to medication will pump and discard the breast milk when the medication is at peak level in the mother's blood. You can ask your prescribing clinician for guidance about this procedure which requires planning ahead to save breast milk and establishing a good breastfeeding routine for you and your baby.

If you are breastfeeding, there are some medications to avoid, such as the benzodiazepines used for anxiety and stimulants used for attention deficit disorders. If you are advised to wean your baby off your own breast milk, in order to take medication, remember the goal is to have both a happy, healthy baby *and* mom—and many babies do just fine with formula.

Costs of Medications

The prices of medications vary in different parts of the country and even in different pharmacies in the same town. To find the best price, shop around. You may find it less expensive to use a mail-order pharmacy. However, one disadvantage of a mail-order pharmacy is that it may be inconvenient to order repeatedly if your dose changes frequently.

Clinicians can sometimes give you samples of a medication to see if you can tolerate it well or if it is even effective for you. The newer medications are more likely to be available as samples. Ask the prescribing clinician about this option.

Some drug companies have programs for people on low incomes, providing medication free or at low cost. These companies usually require the physician or nurse to complete a form and for you to provide proof of your income. If, for budget reasons, you cannot afford these medications, ask your prescribing clinician about this option.

More Research Needed

Over the past twenty years, researchers have collected information about the use of medications in pregnant and postpartum women. We know much more now than we have in years past about the effects of medications on a baby. Still, many women are adamantly opposed to taking medication during and after pregnancy.

It may be helpful for new mothers to know that in 2015, the Food and Drug Administration released a new safety rating system for drugs. Under the new system, pharmaceutical companies must label all drugs, listing the pros and cons of taking the drug for pregnant women and those who are breastfeeding. It is required that any medication approved after June 2001 include this safety information; this gives clinicians a much better guide to prescribing medications.

Still, we have little research to guide us. Very few clinical trials have been conducted on women who are breastfeeding. Further research is needed on the specific short- and long-term effects of medications for pregnant and postpartum women and their babies.

Follow-Up with Your Therapist

After a treatment plan has been formulated, you will generally have a follow-up scheduled with your mental health professional within One to three weeks, depending on the treatment. Be sure you have contact information of the mental health professional and know how to reach his or her office if you have questions. Many offices have e-mail options that may be convenient for asking questions or seeking clarification. Sometimes, if medication is prescribed, the clinician will want to hear from you before your next follow-up visit.

Non-Medication Treatments

For some women, especially those with mild to moderate depression, there are some non-pharmacological treatment options that may be considered. Be aware that the evidence of effectiveness for these treatments is not robust. I would recommend that you consult with a health care provider who can help you assess whether these treatments are appropriate for you.

Psychotherapy

Of all the non-medication treatments, *psychotherapy* is probably used the most. Many pregnant women, whose depression is in the mild range, need increased emotional support and psychotherapy, which may help alleviate symptoms enough to delay further treatment until after delivery. As explained earlier, therapies for depression and anxiety can include supportive, interpersonal, and cognitive-behavioral therapy.

If psychotherapy is your initial choice of treatment, caution must be paid to making sure you are not minimizing mood and anxiety symptoms. If therapy is not sufficient and your symptoms are moderate or severe, consideration must be given to medication. If a woman comes to see me and is adamantly opposed to medication, then I will likely offer therapy with the understanding that if her symptoms do not improve, we need to discuss medication.

I usually like to involve the family if possible in order to educate them also about an illness and to discuss how to be supportive. Often, the family's relationship will provide a trusting environment to allow education and a frank discussion of the risks and benefits of medication. Sometimes, however, family members are opposed to medication and unduly influence the decision about medication. Of course, the ultimate decision always lies with the mother and her partner.

In a study of 4,000 women who gave birth during the course of a year, 67 percent of them had chosen to take medication during pregnancy. The researchers for this study argue that more therapy options for the mother and her partner may help reduce the impact of the illness and may be helpful in avoiding medication use. These researchers believe that therapy provides social support, buoys hope, and helps "mobilize" a woman's own problem-solving to help her feel better. There are currently several valuable studies about the effectiveness of group therapy, but more are needed.

Light Therapy

The use of light has been a treatment option for depression for many years, particularly in people who are affected by seasonal variations in light.

Light therapy is exposure to a certain light range of 7-10, 00 LUX for a time period every morning. It is believed that this treatment may be beneficial for pregnant and postpartum women for several reasons. Some women may have less exposure to light, either because they are pregnant and less mobile, or because they are trying to sleep during the day after having a baby. (Low light is around 1-2000 LUX.) Additionally, the lack of sleep and accompanying fatigue that accompanies having a baby may disrupt the major neurotransmitter system of the brain which controls mood and anxiety—the serotonin system. Light therapy may help regulate the system and may help improve mood.

Hormonal changes may disrupt the serotonin system and exposure to light may help. There is also some evidence that women who have babies in the fall or winter have more risk of postpartum depression because of diminished light exposure at that time of year. A new mother named Donetta describes how light therapy worked for her:

I planned my pregnancy very carefully, because I have had severe depression most of my life. I stopped taking my medication two months before I got pregnant. I was somewhat depressed in the first two trimesters, but in the third I became very depressed, extremely anxious, suicidal, and I could not sleep or eat. I did not want to take any medication, so my psychiatrist suggested I try light therapy. I used the light box three times a week, and it seemed to help. I was still depressed, but it helped me sleep and be less anxious. I was able to delay taking medication until right after delivery.

Light therapy is convenient, can be done at home, and is not expensive. It presents few risks to the fetus. However, light therapy may not work for everyone. In some people, light therapy can cause mood swings or may cause agitation or racing thoughts.

If you have bipolar disorder or have mood swings, do not use this treatment without discussing it with your health care provider. If your mood symptoms are severe, your clinician will likely agree that this is not a treatment option for you.

Over-the-Counter Supplements

Some people have found that taking some over-the-counter supplements are helpful in treating mild to moderate depression. Early studies found that there may be a positive effect in perinatal psychiatry, but not many recent studies have been done for this population, so I am not convinced this is a viable option for treatment or prevention. There may even be some risk if bipolar disorder is present.

Fatty Acids. Fatty acids, such as omega oils, ", and others, have been studied to see if these compounds can be of use in prevention or treatment of perinatal mood disorders. However, the metabolism and effect of these compounds in the body is complex and not completely understood. At this point, they may play a role as supplements but they are not thought to be of significant help on their own. The risks seem low in their use, and these oils may be a helpful addition to a treatment plan.

SAMe Supplements. More recently, there was hope that the synthetic supplement called *SAMe* would be effective for treating depression. SAMe is a synthetic version of a naturally occurring substance in the body that helps the body make chemicals essential for mood regulation. However, SAMe is not useful for anything but mild depression. Many people mistakenly think it is safe because it is "natural," but the form found is health food stores is a synthetic imitation. Because it is a supplement, it is not scrutinized or regulated by the FDA. There are no studies evaluating safety in pregnancy or lactation. Some potential serious interactions and side effects have been documented, so SAMe should not be used without medical supervision.

Folate. Folate supplementation has been shown to be beneficial for many people with major depressive disorder. Folate is a type of vitamin B; it helps in cell growth and metabolism, and is often prescribed to pregnant women. It has been widely used prior to birth to prevent birth defects.

Currently, many clinicians do genetic testing to see if a folate supplement is appropriate for you. If you have chronic depression, talk to your health care provider about adding a pharmaceutical-grade folate to your treatment plan; it may help but is not likely to be effective as a stand-alone treatment.

Electroconvulsive Therapy

A controversial yet relatively safe treatment for depression is *electroconvulsive therapy (ECT)*. This treatment is used for pregnant and postpartum women whose depression has not responded to medication or who cannot take medication. It consists of a series of electrical shocks to the brain while the patient is under anesthesia. Unfortunately, this treatment has a stigma attached to it because of negative depictions in the media—most of us have seen "shock treatments" as they were given years ago—with the patient convulsing in pain.

However, modern-day ECT bears no resemblance to the early version of ECT. Nowadays, it is administered in a way that causes no pain. In addition to being under anesthesia, a patient is given a muscle relaxant. After a treatment, a patient will feel sleepy and probably will not remember what happened for a while. ECT is recommended only when all other options are unsuccessful. A comprehensive review of the use of ECT during pregnancy concludes that ECT during all trimesters in pregnancy is safe and should be considered a valid treatment option. If ECT has been recommended, keep an open mind, seek consultation, and educate yourself about this treatment.

Support Groups

Another popular non-medication treatment is a support group, especially in locales large enough to support an ongoing group of women with a peer-led support group format. Postpartum Support International (listed in the Resource section in the back of the book) provides some guidance in the development of these groups as well as education about depression and anxiety for lay and professional providers.

The support groups offer important benefits to the pregnant or postpartum woman. First of all, they offer a sense that the woman is not alone. Many women feel a stigma at having mood or anxiety symptoms, and often feel a sense of shame or of being a failure. Support groups can offer stories of women with similar symptoms as well as offer practical and helpful support about how to cope, how to deal with families, and how to access the health care system. This information can make a big difference to a woman who is having mood or anxiety problems.

Ann Smith, R.N., a certified nurse midwife and current president of Postpartum Support International, believes "the most important thing about peer support groups is for moms going through postpartum depression to be able to look into the eyes of someone else who is also experiencing depression and not feel so alone and stigmatized." Ms. Smith has run support groups for ten years, and found them invaluable to women.

What Can I Do to Help Myself?

There are a few lifestyle changes you can make on your own that can help improve how you feel. Exercise has been found to help some people with mild to moderate depression stabilize or improve their mood. Although studies have not been conducted specifically with postpartum women, we can safely assume that the effects will be the same for both groups of women. Exercise has proved to be the most effective strategy in changing a "bad" mood into a positive mood when compared to other useful self-help strategies such as socializing, distraction, and relaxation techniques.

Routine Exercise

The positive effect of exercise on women's self-esteem was demonstrated in a study of twenty-seven female volunteers who were not clinically depressed. These volunteers participated in an eight-week walking program. It is not clear whether the exercise must be vigorous or whether a more moderate approach, such as walking, is just as effective. The women reported an increase in positive self-esteem.

Postpartum women have several reasons to exercise. It provides physical conditioning after pregnancy that will help the body return to its pre-pregnant state. It will help improve the overall health of women who are already stressed due to a lack of sleep. Physical activity helps promote sleep.

If you are depressed, you may find it harder to make yourself exercise. Having a friend or another mother join you may help motivate you until the exercise routine becomes a habit. A scheduled exercise time that is a preplanned part of your daily routine will help reinforce your decision to exercise. Although the effects are not dramatic and quick, over time you will notice that you feel better, you have more energy, and your mood is brighter.

Some people with severe depression or bipolar disorder can sometimes use intense regular exercise, along with medications, to manage their mood. However, specific application of exercise as a treatment for mood and anxiety symptoms in pregnancy and postpartum has not yielded significant results. A study in Norway examined women who were at risk for depression; researchers found that starting a program of exercise during pregnancy did not help women who were depressed in the postpartum period.

One caution about exercise: many consumer websites promote exercise as something you can do to help your mood. If done properly, exercise is not going to negatively impact a

106

fetus or a nursing baby. However, may women may start an intense exercise program after delivery; then, if they start having symptoms of postpartum depression or anxiety, they may stop the exercise program. This likely contributes to a sense of failure. Exercise can have a positive effect, but for moderate-to severe symptoms, it is unlikely to help enough that the woman doesn't need clinical treatment.

Good Nutrition

Good nutrition is essential for everyone, but it is especially important for people with mood disorders. Excessive amounts of sugar can cause mood changes severe enough to affect your work or concentration. Caffeine can trigger both anxiety and mood changes, so it should be avoided. Alcohol and other drugs can affect mood adversely and can affect the level of medications present in your body. If taken at all, alcohol should be used in only moderate amounts, such as one or two drinks per week.

Other Strategies

Research has been done on other mood-regulating strategies for both men and women. Besides proper exercise and nutrition, socializing techniques such as talking to others, being with people, and even talking on the phone may help. Distracting techniques such as listening to music, doing housework, and watching TV or reading are used by some people. Another strategy that may be useful is to give yourself a "pep talk" or remind yourself of all the positive aspects of your life. What are you grateful for? Feeling gratitude is a good tool for helping you feel "in the present." Passive techniques such as napping or sleeping are helpful to some people.

There are some activities that you should avoid—activities that may cause you to spiral downward into an emotional slump. These include: isolating yourself, using alcohol to escape your feelings, or blaming yourself for your mood.

9

Help for
Fathers and Families

My wife got depressed just before the baby was born. I was scared, but I thought everything would be okay when the baby got here. No one could have convinced me that my wife would become very depressed, suicidal, not interested in the baby. She was also withdrawn from me. I remember living for about a month in terror that my wife would never be the same. I feared that I would lose the love of my life and have to take care of our new baby by myself.

My wife did recover from her depression. Now, my daughter is almost three, and my wife wants another baby. I don't think I can go through that again, not even for another wonderful child.

Mark, new father

Mark's story illustrates the trauma a new father may experience if his wife becomes severely depressed. The unexpected problems frightened Mark so much that he is reluctant to consider having another baby. Postpartum depression drastically affects not only the new mother but also the new father. Even though health care providers are aware that husbands, fathers, and partners may be affected, most clinicians probably don't realize how many fathers experience depression after the birth of their baby. *The Journal of Advanced Nursing* reports that when women are having symptoms of postpartum depression, as many as 24 to 50 percent of their male partners may also be experiencing depression.

This information clearly compels health care providers to assess the family unit, especially the husband/partner of a woman with perinatal psychiatric problems. At this point, there is not a specific screening tool for men like the Edinburgh Postnatal Depression Scale for women. Until there is such a tool for men, paying attention to the couple and the potential risk for new fathers needs to be a part of good treatment.

Risk Factors for Depression in New Fathers

Following are several factors that may increase a new father's risk for depression:

Feeling Ignored

Too often, fathers take the "backseat" during pregnancy and after the baby arrives. The focus is on the baby and the mother. As a result, the new father may feel left out. When the new mother has problems with depression or anxiety, the father's emotions may be overlooked. He is expected to "take care of things" while his wife recovers. There may be little support or education for the father going through such a crisis.

Previous Loss

Just as a previous loss of a baby in pregnancy or infancy is a risk factor for women, it is also a risk factor for fathers. Sometimes with a miscarriage, for example, the focus is on the mother and her grief, while fathers are often ignored. Often, the couple does not grieve in the same manner, and this can lead to conflict within a couple's relationship.

Feeling Helpless about Wife's Depression

When a pregnant woman or new mother is depressed or having problems with anxiety, a new father is often stressed about his wife's health; he's often also stressed over having increased responsibilities in caring for her and the baby. Research shows that postpartum fathers experience frustration at "not being able to fix the problem." I have heard many new fathers make this statement. This sense of powerlessness leads to fear, confusion, and helplessness.

Medical researchers suggest that health care providers become more aware of the impact a new mother's psychiatric illness can have on her partner. New dads often need more support.

Problems with the Baby and Marital Conflict

Another important factor affecting new fathers is having a difficult child or perhaps a child with medical problems. Again, the sense of worry and helplessness that a parent experiences when their child is ill can be overwhelming. Another important stressor can be an existing marital conflict. Parenting is hard enough when you have a good relationship with your partner, but when the partners are not getting along well, the stress level increases.

Lack of Sleep

The lack of sleep that comes with a new baby can negatively affect the father's mood, especially if he is working as well as taking care of the infant and his wife. All of this can add up to a sense of being fatigued and overwhelmed.

I'm a New Father—Why Am I So Angry?

You may be angry for many reasons. You are under a tremendous amount of stress. You are likely suffering from lack of sleep, which can affect your coping skills. You may feel pressured to juggle responsibilities at home and at work. In addition, even though you are trying to be understanding, you may feel that your wife has let you down. After all, no one wants to be solely responsible for an infant. In essence, you and your wife had a "contract"—it may be that she would take care of the baby while you provided the income, or that you both would work and share in the baby's care. Yet, because of her illness you may feel as if your wife is not living up to her end of the bargain. Be patient and help support her emotionally and practically until she feels better. Only then can she do her part.

What Can a New Father Do?

Sometimes, men worry that their relationships with their wives will never be the same as before the birth of their child. Your wife, naturally, is focused on the baby. Keep in mind, though, that she isn't rejecting you. Mother Nature has helped our species survive by providing women with intensely focused mothering behaviors, necessary for the helpless infant's survival. As the baby gets older, her intense focus on the baby will lessen.

However, if your wife is having problems with depression or anxiety after childbirth, your concerns may be even greater. Although you may be accustomed to facing problems together, for now you may not be able to rely on her to help

110

you. Despite this loss of your wife's usual coping mechanisms, she will get better. It may be helpful for you to think of the current crisis as a temporary situation. With the treatments available today, you can be optimistic that your wife will once again be your partner. Returning to her old self may take longer than you think it should, but the following are ways to help.

Be Supportive

First of all, listen to the mother of your child without criticizing or judging. You may not understand what is happening, but neither does she. It will be very helpful to her to be able to talk openly with you. Also, realize she may feel guilty about her lack of interest in normal activities at this time. Reassure her that you believe she will soon be like herself again.

Get Involved

Participate in the new mother's treatment as much as you can. Educate yourself about postpartum disorders—don't rely on guesswork. Go with your wife to appointments so you can meet the people who are helping her. Understand why a particular treatment has been recommended. Most of all, support your wife in whatever treatment plan she chooses. Even if you aren't comfortable with the therapist or don't like the idea of your wife taking medication, follow her lead.

If a new mother feels comfortable with her therapist and with using medications, try not to undermine her efforts by criticizing or disagreeing with the plan of care. Don't ask for details after every therapy session. Let her know you are interested and want to hear only whatever she feels comfortable sharing. Therapy sessions are often very intense, so it may take her a while to formulate her thoughts.

Do More at Home or Get Help

You may need to take on more than your share of responsibility for the baby and the house. Reprioritize your social and work commitments so you will have more time and energy. Taking on this kind of responsibility may be a brand-new experience, for which you may not be prepared. But you can do it with the help and advice from family and friends. Realize that your wife will eventually be able to take on her part, but right now she simply can't.

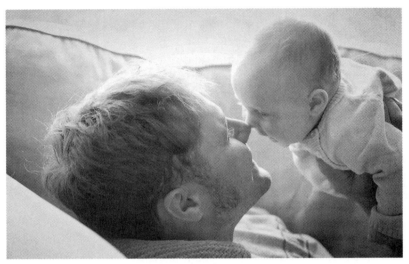

According to researchers, depression in new fathers is underscreened, underdiagnosed, and undertreated. Depression in either parent can prevent them from engaging in tender caregiving, which in turn, can affect a baby's mood.

If you do not have time off available from work, you may want to consider taking time off under the *Family and Medical Leave Act of 1993.* You may be eligible to take time to help your wife and baby without it affecting your position at work. There are some restrictions to this policy, though, so be sure to check with your employer's human resources department or benefit administrator.

Act as a Mediator with Extended Families

You may need to educate both of your extended families about what is happening. Help them understand that their advice, criticism, or judgmental comments will not help your wife right now. Chances are, family members who are critical do not know about or understand postpartum mood disorders. You can also suggest to them practical ways in which they may be able to help both you and your wife.

Seek Help for Yourself, Too

These steps to help your wife may leave you feeling exhausted, resentful, and overwhelmed. Don't be critical of yourself as a new father. Under the circumstances, your feelings are normal.

If you need someone to help you at this time, consider seeking therapy for yourself. Having someone aware of what you are going through will help you provide better support for your wife. Unfortunately, there are few support systems, such as support groups, designed for new fathers or partners. Ask other husbands or partners if their wives had problems after delivery. Chances are, you will hear experiences from other fathers that will help you feel less alone.

This difficult time may cause distance between you and your spouse at a time when you most need to work closely together. If the two of you need marital counseling, arrange for couple's counseling so that you can both air these feelings and renew your partnership, both as a couple and as parents. The following story from thirty-three-year-old Delain illustrates how the marital relationship can be affected by postpartum anxiety:

> After the baby came, I had to go back to work after taking one week off to be at home. I was feeling this incredible sense of responsibility and felt unprepared to be a father.
>
> My wife started having panic attacks when left alone. I was very angry at her. I thought she was being unreasonable. I felt betrayed by her, like she was leaving me with all the responsibility of the baby, her health, and earning a living! We fought the whole weekend before I was to go back to work. On Sunday, she told me she wanted to kill herself. That scared me so much I called the doctor who delivered the baby. He said, "Sounds like she is having postpartum depression." I was shocked. I didn't know this could happen.
>
> I took my wife to see a therapist who explained my wife had an anxiety disorder and recommended therapy and medication. We got a baby-sitter for the daytime, and after about two weeks, my wife was so much better. I met with her therapist to talk about how I was feeling, and that helped. We are back to our good relationship and having a good time with the baby. I am so grateful for the attention we paid to our relationship, not just her anxiety.

Delain's feelings about his wife's illness are normal, and choosing the right time and place to express them is important. Just as he experienced relief in talking with someone about how he felt, doing so may prove helpful for you, too. Find a therapist or health care provider who you feel comfortable with and who is knowledgeable about postpartum mood disorders.

Even though you both wanted this baby, seeing your wife experience depression or anxiety as a result of having a child may stir up feelings of guilt. Keep in mind that you are not responsible for your wife's condition. But you can help her through her treatment so that you can both enjoy being parents as well as partners.

A Father's Concern about Safety

Although most women pose no risk to themselves or their baby, your wife may be so ill that her judgment is impaired. If so, you will need to take action immediately. If she is talking about hurting herself or the baby, take her immediately to an emergency room. Do not leave her alone. If she is agitated, having delusions or hallucinations, treat this behavior as a medical emergency and seek medical help immediately.

Father-Baby Relationship

Focusing on the importance of an infant's attachment to the father is a relatively new concept. Prior to 1970, little research had been done about father-infant or father-child relationships. Since then, though, researchers have discovered that infants attach to the people with whom they come into contact. A child's attachment to both the mother and father cannot be emphasized enough as a key factor in the infant's development, both physically and mentally.

Ronnie's view of how he was going to interact with his baby changed quickly when he had to assume the role of primary caretaker:

When my wife had panic attacks and depression after our son was born, I had to take care of the baby most of the time because she couldn't. I had no clue what I was supposed to do. I had thought I would just play with the baby and love it. I didn't know about feeding, bathing, and the amount of care an infant needs. I got help from several people and I read books, but mostly I learned from taking care of the baby.

This was not my original view of what being a father would be like, but now I cherish the time I had to bond with our new baby. I was even a bit jealous when my wife got better and could take care of him more. But I know I am closer to my son because of the time we spent together.

After ten months, my life is almost like it was before the baby came and my wife got depressed—at least as normal as it can be with a toddler! I no longer wake up scared that things will not be alright. I worry some that my wife will get depressed again. I don't know if we will have another baby.

Ronnie's story illustrates the results of successful treatment—his wife got better and his family is back to normal. He will probably always have some worry about his wife, but it no longer dominates his life. It's normal for him to have concerns about future pregnancies, and he and his wife will want to give serious consideration to having additional children.

Decide What Type of Father You Want to Be

Our society has gender-based expectations about parenting. Women are expected to know automatically what to do, while men often take a secondary role. This division of caretaking roles has a historical basis. The traditional father was a breadwinner and a disciplinarian. When household duties were assigned by gender, women took care of the house and the children.

When gender roles began to change and women started working more often outside the home, too, their home-based roles did not change as quickly. Even now, research suggests that fathers are typically involved with their children through such activities as sports, while the primary caretaking role is still left to the mother, regardless of whether she is employed outside the home.

It is hard to know for certain how much of this separation of roles is based on tradition. But child care need not be based on the gender of the parent. In reality, some men have stronger nurturing skills than some women, so they make better primary caretakers. If you are assuming more responsibility for the baby than you thought you would, look on this time as an opportunity to experience a connection with your infant that otherwise might not have occurred.

Some Family Members May Be Affected

Finally, as we have learned more about the prevalence of postpartum depression in fathers, we also need to realize that other family members may be affected emotionally by the arrival of a baby. Any number of past memories of a family member may surface "out of the blue" for them. For example, a family member who has lost a child through miscarriage or early death may find feelings of grief surfacing. And, occasionally, a family member may have totally unexpected thoughts—similar to those of some new mothers—about hurting the baby. Paul, a fifty-nine year old grandfather, remembers his frightening experience:

> My wife and I were so thrilled when we learned our daughter-in-law was pregnant with our first grandchild—a little girl. The entire family was "over the moon" with excitement. However, soon after our granddaughter was born, I was realized I was afraid to be alone with the baby. Even now, these words are hard to say, but: I feared I would hurt her.
>
> I knew deep inside that I would never hurt the baby, but the thoughts were so horrifying that I never told anyone about them. I was deeply ashamed of such insidious thoughts, and I knew I would scare family members if I told them. As our grandchild got older, those ugly thoughts faded away.
>
> Years later, I had a chance to speak to an expert on postpartum depression issues; she said it is fairly common for other family members—aunts, uncles, and grandparents—to have those thoughts, and that they were the type of thoughts that, although scary, are not the type of psychotic thoughts that cause some people to actually take action. I was so relieved to hear this; having talked to her helped me shed some of my shame all these years later.

Family members such as Paul will likely never tell anyone about their frightening thoughts of hurting the baby. But if you know of family members who are avoiding being alone with a new baby or who have expressed these kinds of fears, reassure them that, because they understand how unrealistic their thoughts are, they are not dangerous to the baby, they will not act on those ugly thoughts, and, in reality, they have only deep love for the baby.

10

Looking Ahead

As you begin to feel better, you will probably find yourself starting to think about the future. Indeed, this response indicates your perspective is not focused entirely on how you feel right now. But before we discuss the future, let's take a look at where you have been.

You emerge from the first year after giving birth, having been traumatized by a psychiatric disorder. No doubt, you recall the feelings of guilt, shame, and failure you felt. You probably also remember the sense of isolation you experienced and the frantic search for someone who knew how to treat perinatal psychiatric disorders. Your family was likely traumatized also, and the legacy of the depression, anxiety, or psychosis and its effect on them can last a long time.

If you're like most women, you will long remember the psychiatric problems you experienced during pregnancy and after. I have had many patients in their fifties, sixties, and seventies who recounted their experiences, and their universal statement has been: "I wish I would have had information about psychiatric disorders when I was pregnant or postpartum."

Arlene is a sixty-seven-year-old woman whose story is very typical of women looking back on their experiences:

> When I was twenty-two, I felt so good during my pregnancy, but after the baby was born, I became very depressed. I found myself detached and wanting to avoid the baby. I thought it was because I was not a good mother, or maybe I didn't like babies. My family thought it was because my husband was so enamored of the baby that I was jealous.

This was in the 1970s, and postpartum depression was not as recognized as it is today. But now I realize I was depressed and anxious. Looking back at my childhood, I also realize I had depression and anxiety as a teenager, but I didn't know what to call it. I was never diagnosed or treated. However, having been on medication for many years, I am pleased to say I am doing well.

And, it has been so gratifying to immediately have fallen in love with my granddaughters when they were born. Their births were so different for me compared to when my own children were born. It confirms for me I was a good mother, and I loved my children—I was just depressed.

As you think about the depression or anxiety that has affected you so profoundly, you may find yourself fearful that it will happen again. Most people who have been depressed or affected by severe anxiety dread a recurrence to such an extent that even a slight depression, a bad day, or a period of anxiety may stir up their fears. They may even assume they are "back where they started."

But getting better is a gradual process with ups and downs along the way. As you recover, you can anticipate having fewer and fewer bad days, but you will still have some. If you are having a slump after several good days or weeks, do not "catastrophize" or exaggerate the significance of briefly feeling somewhat like you did before. Juli reacted strongly to increased anxiety and feared she was going to relapse:

For about three weeks, I was feeling so good that I thought I was completely cured of my postpartum anxiety. Even though my therapist had told me that I would have problems with anxiety again, I secretly told myself I was never going to feel that way again.

But one morning, I woke up feeling this ball of anxiety in my stomach, just like I used to. Crying, I panicked and called my husband, "It's happening again!" I said. He came home and was very worried. He called my therapist and scheduled an emergency session.

By that afternoon I was feeling better, but went to the therapist. I learned I was unrealistic about never having anxiety again. I had to learn to monitor and manage my anxiety. I felt some anger and sadness about having this problem in my life, but fortunately there were medications available and people who understood. Now when I have a bad day, I make sure I get plenty of sleep, decrease my stress, and ask for help from my husband and friends.

Juli's unrealistic belief that she was completely over her anxiety is not an uncommon reaction. Whenever an illness occurs that profoundly disrupts our lives, we hope it will never recur. Adjusting to the idea that depression and anxiety may be an ongoing problem can be worrisome.

Now that you are feeling better, you may feel like doing further reading or research about other strategies to help maintain your better mood or calmness. For example, during the early phase of treatment, you may not have felt like going to a support group. But now might be a good time to meet other people with similar problems and learn from them.

Most women who develop symptoms of depression in the perinatal period get better. After about twelve to fifteen months after delivery, the majority of women will report that they are "back to normal" even though they may still be on medication. However, there are some women whose depressive symptoms do not improve. One study describes reports that a significant risk factor for women who do not seem to be getting better is having a partner who is not supportive or who is critical and controlling.

Additionally, an episode of depression prior to pregnancy or a history of a bipolar illness, significant anxiety, or OCD may increase the likelihood that it will take longer to recover. Other factors include persistent stressors, such as financial difficulties, and problems with the health of the mother or baby. You may need a different treatment strategy for you to get well. Pay attention to how you are feeling and if you are not getting better it is important to seek help; if the depression continues for several years, you may be at risk for developing chronic persistent depression.

I'm Better, but My Family Still Worries

As you begin to improve, you may notice that your family shows signs of the stress that has been affecting them. It is not uncommon for families who have been coping well to "fall apart" later, after the new mother has recovered. You may notice your husband becoming more withdrawn or angry, or your other children may start exhibiting unusual behaviors. This normal readjustment period allows them to express their worry, anger, and fear that you will become ill again.

Talk to them about their reactions openly and try to allow them to describe their feelings without trying to fix the situation. Their recovery may be a bit behind yours. They may still be very wary and watchful for signs that you are still ill. Here's what happened in Camilla's family:

> After I started feeling better, my mother and my husband were still very protective. They wouldn't let me drive very far or take the baby out by myself. When I got irritated, they tried to quiet me and tell me not to get upset.
>
> Finally, I told them that I was better and that they needed to loosen up. They both cried and said they were so worried about me; they didn't want me to get depressed again. My therapist suggested that I tell them they don't need to worry so much because I have others who will help me monitor how I am feeling. This talk helped a lot. Now they treat me normally, not like an invalid.

Should I Tell Others about My Postpartum Problems?

Now that you are out and about more, telling friends and family about your depression or anxiety may be stressful. During the acute or severe part of your illness, your focus was on getting treatment and feeling better. Now that you are feeling better, it is up to you to decide how much information you wish to share about your illness with others.

Many new mothers feel a sense of shame and blame themselves for having problems that other mothers may not have. This may inhibit you from wanting to tell others about any emotional problems you've had since the birth of your baby. Still it's important that you seek emotional support, so you may wish to talk to a therapist or a clinician about the feelings you're experiencing. Remember the advice of Dr. Cheryl Beck, a nurse researcher in the field of perinatal psychiatry, "My message to the mothers: you are not weak. You have done nothing wrong and it is not your fault. These disorders are common after delivery, and they are very treatable."

Your Future Pregnancies

If you experienced depression or anxiety during a previous pregnancy, you are at risk of a recurrence with future pregnancies. If you are pregnant and find yourself feeling as you did during your previous pregnancy, seek help immediately. Lorraine, a twenty-nine-year-old, describes her anxiety during three pregnancies:

> I had my first episode of anxiety during my first pregnancy when I was about ten weeks pregnant. I couldn't sleep. I thought I was dying at times. My doctor referred me to a therapist who was very helpful.
>
> After the baby arrived, I thought the panic might come back, but it didn't. However, the panic did return during my next two pregnancies. The last time, I had to use medication to help control the symptoms during the last trimester. I have had these problems only when I was pregnant.

Understand that Each Pregnancy Is Unique

Even though you may be at risk for another episode of depression or anxiety during your pregnancy or after your delivery, your previous experience does not absolutely mean you will have trouble again. Each pregnancy is different. Your mind and body are different now. And, now that you have had some experience with treatment, keep in mind that if you do become depressed or anxious again, seeking early treatment is better than trying to ride it out on your own. In addition to treatment, there are many things you can do yourself. Take care of yourself and try to stay physically healthy: get enough sleep, eat nutritious meals, and exercise. Taking good care of yourself isn't easy if you have young children, but it is not impossible.

If you decide to have another child, it may be helpful to wait at least two years so that you do not have more than one infant to care for at the same time. Be sure to tell all of your caregivers about your previous episode of postpartum depression or anxiety. Talk with your therapist early in your pregnancy about a treatment plan in case you develop symptoms again. Sometimes, medication may be started immediately after delivery to ward off an episode of depression. Many women have found this very effective.

Don't Isolate Yourself

Make sure that your social needs are met. Connections with other people are vital to both your physical and mental health. To prosper and grow, our relationships need careful attention. Don't focus all of your energy on your family. You need some space for your own interests and time alone or with your friends. Taking care of your needs does not mean that

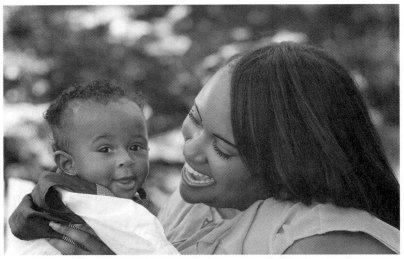

Remember, we don't usually find happiness—we bring it into our lives. Take care of your emotional needs and stay socially connected. Happy mothers usually have happy babies.

you are being selfish. Don't say "yes" to everyone else and "no" to yourself. A major part of taking care of yourself is being sure that you have some fun in your own life. What do you do for fun? If the only answer you have is collapsing in front of the TV after putting your children to bed, then perhaps you need to develop other outlets for yourself.

Minimize Stress

Develop a plan to minimize the stress in your life. Perhaps you can put off that remodeling job or the move to a bigger house for a while. If you have gone back to work, make a conscious effort not to overextend yourself. For many young families, finances are a major source of stress. Perhaps a consultation with a financial planner can help ease your stress about money.

Nurture Your Relationships

Don't neglect the relationship with your husband or partner. Be sure to spend time alone as a couple so that you reconnect as adults who fell in love, when it was just the two of you. You need to nurture your relationship now because someday it will be just the two of you again, and you don't want to be strangers.

Watch for Early Warning Signs

By now you probably recognize the signs that you are getting anxious or depressed. Perhaps you've not slept well for several weeks, or you are sleeping too much. Maybe you notice that you don't want to leave the house. Do you notice that you feel irritable and get angry over small issues? Often, recognizing early signs and paying attention to them can head off another episode. If the symptoms persist, call your therapist. Paying attention to the balance in your life and correcting any "tilts" will help. Remember that achieving balance is a process. If you get out of balance, it doesn't mean you are back to where you started, it just means that you need to do whatever is necessary to help regain your equilibrium.

Efforts to Prevent Postpartum Disorders

Research is ongoing for finding ways to treat and prevent postpartum psychiatric disorders. Numerous forms of preventive measures have been studied, but unfortunately, none of them has been widely useful. For example, because it is thought that hormonal imbalances might be a cause of postpartum psychiatric disorders, medical researchers believed treating women with hormones before they gave birth might help; this was helpful in preventing postpartum disorders in some women, but the practice was not useful to a great number of women.

One research survey involved women taking the antidepressant *nortiptyline* as a preventive measure. Unfortunately, this study concluded that using the antidepressant was not that helpful.

Another scientific study looked at giving women supplemental folic acid, an enzyme that can play a role in regulating moods; however, this study provided no promising results for most women.

Additional research looked at a possible link between inflammation and depression and anxiety disorders. As you know, inflammation involves redness, swelling, and pain after an injury, such as an insect bite or a cut to the finger. However, there is also a type of inflammation that can affect the entire body.

Eating Placenta: Not Recommended

The practice of a new mother eating her placenta after she's given birth is called *placentophagy*. (The placenta is processed and prepared for consumption—sometimes it's dried, ground into powder, and made into capsules.) Advocates believe that because many mammals eat their placentas, perhaps women should as a way to prevent postpartum depression. However, animals eat their placentas after delivery for nutritional purposes, to clean their nests, and to rid the nesting area of any scents that could attract predators.

According to the journal *Scientific American,* this practice is a "growing fad," and there is *no evidence that it is beneficial for a woman to eat her placenta.* Further, there is risk of infection if a contaminant such as meconium stool is present. Meconium, the first bowel movement of a newborn, is composed of materials ingested by the fetus while in the uterus.

Research on how inflammation may contribute to postpartum disorders is ongoing along with numerous other studies.

Need for Screening and Education

Postpartum depression is one of the few illnesses in psychiatry for which we have some ability to predict which women are more at risk. For more than twenty years, we have known of postpartum disorder risk factors such as:

- previous episode of depression or anxiety
- previous diagnosis of bipolar disorder
- major threats to the health of mother or baby
- a previous pregnancy/infant loss
- major changes in the life situation such as a death or move
- an abusive relationship
- being a single mother without a high-school education

Any of these factors place a new mother at risk for developing depression and anxiety. Yet there is no systematic, nationwide awareness/education campaign for new mothers and their families. Many obstetricians do not routinely screen women for emotional problems during pregnancy; others wait four to six weeks postpartum to screen, if they do it at all.

The American Academy of Pediatrics recommends screening in the early postpartum period and later. Their study of

2,354 women showed that 13 percent were identified as having postpartum depression.

Unfortunately, all depression in the United States has gone underdiagnosed and undertreated in past years. However, in 2016, a Preventative Task Force, made up of health professionals and experts in depression prevention, made a recommendation intended to increase public awareness about depression. The task force recommended that all adults, including pregnant and postpartum women, be screened for depression; the task force also recommended that systems should be in place to treat those with depression.

You might think of this recommendation as being similar to the one that began years ago, encouraging Americans to undergo colon cancer screening after age fifty. As public awareness grew, more people underwent screenings.

In Summary

It has now been more than one hundred years since Dr. Louis Victor Marcé, the French physician, first categorized postpartum psychiatric problems. He would likely be amazed that we still have so much to learn about these relatively common and predictable disorders. But we have made progress, particularly in the last twenty years. In fact, never before in history have we had access to such advanced medical technology—technology that helps ensure the health and well-being of both mother and child. Whether a mother's needs are physical or emotional, help is available.

If I could make one wish, it would be that in the next few years no one will say to me, "I didn't know about depression or anxiety or the fact either of these could occur during pregnancy or after I had a baby."

Also, there is still a stigma in our society for people with psychiatric symptoms. Despite some progress being made, the stigma for pregnant and new mothers is even more pervasive and women often feel shame and guilt, leading them to hide their symptoms even from their spouses.

There is no reason to suffer in silence and in shame. Seek the support of knowledgeable professionals. Early intervention while you are pregnant is essential to both your health and your baby's health. You can find considerable relief in working with a therapist who is well informed about postpartum psychiatric disorders. The very act of talking to a trusted professional about what you are feeling often helps. You deserve to feel good about this important phase of your life. Try to look at the "big picture"—understand that any depression or anxiety you may be experiencing now is temporary. With proper treatment, you can, indeed, enjoy being a mother.

Bibliography

Chapter 1

Beck C. 2001. Predictors of postpartum depression: An update. *Nursing Research.* 50(5):275.285.

Beydoun H.A., Beydoun M.A., Kaufmann J.S., et al. 2012. Intimate partner violence against adult women and its association with major depressive disorder, depressive symptoms and postpartum depression: A systematic review and meta-analysis. *Social Science and Medicine.* 75:959-975.

Buist A., Barnett B. 1995. Childhood sexual abuse: a risk factor for postpartum depression. *Australian and New Zealand Journal of Psychiatry.* 29:4.

Correspondence with Cheryl Beck, DNSc, CNM, FAAN, Board of Trustees Distinguished Professor, School of Nursing, University of Connecticut, April 24, 2015.

Creasy R.K., Resnik R. 1994. Maternal-fetal medicine: Principles and practice. Philadelphia: W.B. Saunders.

Dix C. 1985. *The New Mother Syndrome.* New York: Pocket Books.

Final Recommendation Statement: Depression in Adults: Screening. U. S. Preventive Services Task Force, January 2016.

Gulamani S.S., Premji S.S., Zeenat Khanu K., Azam S.I. 2013. A Review of Postpartum Depression, Preterm Birth and Culture. *Journal of Perinatal and Neonatal Nursing.* 27(1):52-59.

Hamilton J.A., Harberger P.N., eds. 1992. *Postpartum psychiatric illness: A picture puzzle.* Philadelphia: University of Pennsylvania Press.

Iles S., Gath D., Kennerley H. 1989. Maternity blues: A comparison between post-operative women and post-natal women. *British Journal of Psychiatry.* 155:363-366.

Interview with Steve Machlin, M.D., July 7, 2015.

Kendall, R.E., Chalmers, J.C., Platz, C. 1987. Epidemiology of puerperal psychoses. *British Journal of Psychiatry.* 150:662-673.

Kolte A.M., Olsen L.R., Mikkelsen E.M., Christiansen O.B., Nielsen H.S. 2015. Depression and emotional stress is highly prevalent among women with recurrent pregnancy loss. *Human Reproduction.* 30(4): 777-782.

Matthey S., Barnett B., Howie P., and Kavanaugh D.J. 2003. Diagnosing postpartum depression in mothers and fathers: whatever happened to anxiety? *Journal of Affective Disorders.* 74(2): 139-147.

O'Hara, M.W., Schlechte, J.A., Lewis, D.A., Wright, E.J. 1991. Prospective study of postpartum blues: Biologic and pyschosocial factors. *Archives of General Psychiatry.* 48:801-806.

Rambelli, C., Montagnani, M.S., Oppo, A., et al. 2010. Panic disorder as a risk factor for postpartum depression: Results from the Parenatal Depression-Research & Screening Unit Study. *Journal of Affective Disorders.* 122:139-143.

Chapter 2

Kennerly H., Gath D. 1989. Maternity blues: Associations with obstetric, psychological and psychiatric factors. *British Journal of Psychiatry.* 155:367-373.

O'Hara M.W., et al, eds. 1995. *Psychological aspects of women's reproductive health.* New York: Springer.

Chapter 3

Beck, C.T. 1995. The effects of postpartum depression on maternal-infant interaction: A meta-analysis. *Nursing Research.* 44:5.

Diagnostic and Statistical Manual of Mental Disorders. 2014. 5th Edition. American Psychiatric Association.

Hamilton J.A., Harberger P.N. eds. 1992. *Postpartum psychiatric illness: A picture puzzle.* Philadelphia: University of Pennsylvania Press.

Hay D.F., Kumar R. 1995. Interpreting the effects of mother's postnatal depression on children's intelligence: A critique and re-analysis. *Child Psychiatry and Human Development.* 25 (3):165-181.

Healy B. 1995. *A new prescription for women's health: Getting the best medical care in a man's world.* New York: Penguin.

Jack D.C. 1991. *Silencing the self: Women and depression.* Cambridge, Mass: Harvard University Press.

Maldonado, M. Interview with author. May, 1996.

McGrath E., ed. 1990. Women and depression. Washington, D.C.: *American Psychological Association.*

Bibliography

O'Hara M., et al, eds. 1995. *Psychological aspects of women's reproductive health.* New York: Springer Publishing.

Paffenbarger R.S. 1982. *Epidemiological aspects of mental illness associated with childbearing.* Brockington I.F., Kumar R., eds. Motherhood and mental illness. New York: Grune and Stratton.

Papolos D., Papolos J. 3d ed. 1997. *Overcoming depression.* New
York: Harper Perennial.

Parry B.L. 1989. Reproductive Factors Affecting the Course of Affective Illness in Women. *Psychiatric Clinics of North America.* 12.1:
207-220.

Pauliekhoff B. 1992. Toward the diagnosis of postpartum psychotic
depression. Hamilton, J.A., Harberger P.N., eds. *Postpartum psychiatric illness: A picture puzzle.* Philadelphia: University of Pennsylvania Press.

Sichel D.A., et al. 1995. Prophylactic estrogen in recurrent postpartum affective disorder. *Biological Psychiatry.* 38:814-818.

Stern D. N. 1985. *The interpersonal world of the infant.* New York:
Basic Books.

Stowe Z.N., et al. 1995. Sertraline in the treatment of women with
postpartum major depression. *Depression.* 3:49-55.

Wieck A., et al. 1991. Increased sensitivity of dopamine receptors
and recurrence of affective psychosis after childbirth. *British Medical Journal.* 303 (6803):613-616.

Chapter 4

Amerio, A., Odone, A., Marchesi, C., Ghaemi, S.N., 2014. Treatment
of comorbid bipolar disorder and obsessive compulsive disorder:
a systematic review. *Journal of Affective Disorders.* 166:258-263.

Diagnostic and Statistical Manual of Mental Disorders. 2014. 5th
Edition. American Psychiatric Association.

Miller, E.S., Chu, C., Gollan, J. and Gossett, D.R. 2015. Obsessive-
compulsive symptoms during the postpartum period: A prospective cohort. *Journal of Reproductive Medicine.* March, 2015.

Misri, S. 1995. *Shouldn't I be happy: Emotional problems of pregnant
and postpartum women.* New York: Free Press.

Pallanti, S. and Grassi, G. 2014. Pharmacologic treatment of obsessive-compulsive disorder comorbidity. Expert opinion. *Pharmacotherapy.* 15(17): 2543-2552.

Chapter 5

Andersen L.B., Velvaer L.B., Videbech P., Lamont R.F., Joergensen
J.S. 2012. Risk factors for developing post-traumatic stress disorder
following childbirth: a systematic review. *Acta Obstetricia et Gynecologica Scandinavica.* 91:1261-1271.

Diagnostic and Statistical Manual of Mental Disorders. 2014. 5th Edition. American Psychiatric Association.

Engler J., Goleman D. 1992. *The consumer's guide to psychotherapy*. New York: Simon & Schuster.

Furuta M., Sandall J., and Bick D. 2012. A Systematic review of the relationship between severe maternal morbidity and post-traumatic stress disorder. *BMC Pregnancy and Childbirth*. 12:125.

Karsnitz D.B. Ward S. 2011. Spectrum of anxiety disorder: diagnosis and pharmacologic treatment. *Journal of Midwifery and Women's Health*. 56: 266-281.

Misri, S. 1995. *Shouldn't I be happy: Emotional problems of pregnant and postpartum women*. New York: Free Press.

Somerville, S., Dedman, K., Hagan, R., et al. The Perinatal Anxiety Screening Scale: development and preliminary validation. *Archives of Women's Mental Health*. DOI:10.1007/s00737-014-0425-8.

Chapter 6

Belluck, P. June 15, 2014. Thinking of ways to harm her. *New York Times*.

Diagnostic and Statistical Manual of Mental Disorders. 2014. 5th Edition. American Psychiatric Association.

Doucet, S., Jones, I., Letourneau, N,. Dennis, C., Blackmore, E.R. 2011. Interventions for the treatment and prevention of postpartum psychosis: a systematic review. *Archives of Women's Mental Health*. 14:89-98.

Jones, I., Chandra, P.S., Dazzan, P., Howard, L.M. 2014. Bipolar disorder, affective psychosis, and schizophrenia in pregnancy and postpartum. *The Lancet*. 384:1789-1799.

Pauliekhoff, B. 1992. Toward the diagnosis of postpartum psychotic depression. Hamilton, J.A. and P.N. Harberger, eds. *Postpartum psychiatric illness: A picture puzzle*. Philadelphia: University of Pennsylvania Press.

Sichel, D. A., et al. 1995. Prophylactic estrogen in recurrent postpartum affective disorder. *Biological Psychiatry*. 38:814-818.

Spinelli, M.G. 2009. Postpartum psychosis: detection of risk and management. *American Journal of Psychiatry*. 166:4.

Stahl, S.M. 2001. Natural estrogen as an antidepressant for women. *Journal of Clinical Psychiatry*. 62(6):404-405.

Chapter 7

Andrews, G. et al. 1994. *The treatment of anxiety disorders: Clinician's guide and patient manuals*. New York: Cambridge University Press.

Antonuccio, D.O., W.G. Danton, and G.Y. DeNelsky. 1995. Psycho-

Bibliography

therapy versus medication for depression: Challenging the conventional wisdom with data. *Professional Psychology: Research and Practice.* 26 (6):574-585.

Engler, J. and D. Goleman. 1992. *The consumer's guide to psychotherapy.* New York: Fireside Books.

Meager, I. and J. Milgrom. 1996. Group treatment for postpartum depression: A pilot study. Australian and New Zealand Journal of Psychiatry. 30:852-860.

Mental health: Does therapy help? Consumer Reports. November, 1995.

Miller, I.W., and G.I. Keitner. 1996. *Combined medication and psychotherapy in the treatment of chronic mood disorders.* The Psychiatric Clinics of North America. 19 (1):151-169.

Chapter 8

Altshuler L.L., Cohen L.S., Moline M.L., et al. 2001. *The expert consensus guideline series: treatment of depression in women postgrad medical special report.* March: 1-116.

Brogan K. 2013. *Perinatal depression and anxiety: beyond psychopharmacology.* Psychiatric Clinics of North America. 36:183-188.

Crowley S.K., Youngstedt S.D. (2012). Efficacy of light therapy for perinatal depression: A review *Journal of Physiological Anthropology.* 31

Einarson T.R. and Einarson A. 2005. Newer antidepressants in pregnancy and rates of major malformations: a meta-analysis of prospective comparative studies. *Pharmacoepidemiology and Drug Safety.* 14: 823-827.

Freeman M.P. 2009. Complementary and alternative medicine for perinatal depression. *Journal of Affective Disorders.* 111:1-10.

Goodman S.H., Dimidjian S. 2012. The developmental psychopathology of perinatal depression: Implications for psychosocial treatment development and delivery in pregnancy. *Canadian Journal of Psychiatry.* 57(9):530-536

Gulamani S.S., Premji S.S., Zeenat Khanu K., Azam S.I. 2013. A review of postpartum depression, preterm birth and culture. *Journal of Perinatal and Neonatal Nursing.* 27(1):52-59

Howard L.M., Molyneaux E., Dennis C.L., Rochat T., Stein A., and Milgram J. 2014. Nonpsychotic mental disorders in the perinatal period. *The Lancet.* 384:1775-1788.

Interview with Steve Machlin, M.D. July 7, 2015.

Kim D.R., Epperson C.N., Weiss A. R. and Wisner K. 2014. Pharmacotherapy of postpartum depression: an update. *Expert Opinion, Pharmacotherapy.* 15(9).

Sichel, D.A., et al. 1995. Prophylactic estrogen in recurrent postpartum affective disorder. *Biological Psychiatry*. 38:814-818.

Songøygard K.M., Stafne S.N., Evensen K.A., Salvesen K.Å., Vik T., Mørkved S. (2012). Does exercise during pregnancy prevent postnatal depression? A randomized clinical trial. *Acta Obstetricia et Gynecologica Scandinavica*. Jan:91(1):62-67.

Suri R., Lin A.S.,Cohen L.S., Altshuler L.L. 2014. Acute and long-term behavioral outcome of infants and children exposed in utero to either maternal depression or antidepressants: a review of the literature. *Journal of Clinical Psychiatry*. 75:1143-1152.

Taylor L.G., Thelus J.R., Gordon G., Fram D., Coster T. 2015. Development of a mother-child database for drug exposure and adverse event detection in the military health system. *Pharmacoepidemiology and Drug Safety*. 24: 510-517.

U.S. Food and Drug Administration. www.fda.gov/Drugs/DevelopmentApprovalProcess/DevelopmentResources/Labeling/ucm093307.htm

Vigod S.N., Gomes T., Wilton A.S., Taylor V.H., and Ray J.G. 2015. Antipsychotic drug use in pregnancy: high dimensional, propensity matched, population based cohort study. *British Medical Journal*. 350:h2298.

Walton G.D., Ross L.E., Stewart D.E., et al. 2014. Decisional conflict among women considering antidepressant use in pregnancy. *Archives of Women's Mental Health*. 17:493-501.

Chapter 9

Demontigny F., Girard M.E., Lacharit, C.D., Dubeau D., Devault, A. 2013. Psychosocial factors associated with paternal postnatal depression. *Journal of Affective Disorders*. 15(150):44-49.

Goodman J.H. 2004. Paternal postpartum depression, its relationship to maternal postpartum depression, and implications for family health. *Journal of Advanced Nursing*. 45(1): 26-35.

Lamb, M.E. ed. 1997. *The role of the father in child development*. 3rd ed. New York: John Wiley.

Meighan M., Davis M.W., Thomas S.P, Droppleman G. 1999 Living with postpartum depression: the father's experience. *American Journal of Maternal/Child Nursing*. 24(4): 202-208.

Pinheiro R.T, Magalhaes P.V, Horta L., Pinheiro, K.A., de Silva, R. A, Pinto R.H. 2006. Is paternal postpartum depression associated with maternal postpartum depression? Population-based study in Brazil. *Acta Psychiatrica Scandinavica*. 111(3): 230-232.

Wang S.Y., Chen C.H. 2006. Psychosocial health of Taiwanese postnatal husband and wives. *Journal of Psychosomatic Research*. 60(3): 303-307.

Bibliography

Chapter 10

Beurel E. 2015. A primer on inflammation for psychiatrists. *Psychiatric Annals.* 45(5):226-231.

Boorman E., Romano G.F., Russell A., Mondelli V., Parlante C.M. 2015. Are mood and anxiety disorders inflammatory diseases? *Psychiatric Annals.* 45(5):240-248.

Correspondence with Dr. Cheryl Beck, April 16, 2015.

Harrington R. (2015). Mothers who eat a newborn's placenta may or may not benefit. *Scientific American.* April 2, 2015.

Lewis S J., Araya R., Leary S., Davey Smith, G., Ness A. 2012. Folic acid supplementation during pregnancy may protect against depression 21 months after pregnancy, an effect modified C677 MTHFR C677T genotype. *European Journal of Clinical Nutrition.* 66:97-103.

Sockol L. E., Epperson C.N., Barber J. P. 2013. Preventing postpartum depression: A meta-analytic review. *Clinical Psychology Review.* 33:1205-1217.

Vliegan N., Casalin S., Luyten P. 2014. The course of postpartum depression: A review of longitudinal studies. *Harvard Review of Psychiatry.* 22(1):1-22.

Werner E., Miller M., Osborne, L.M., Kuzava S., Monk C. 2015. Preventing postpartum depression: Review and recommendations. *Archives of Women's Mental Health.* 18:41-60.

Wisner K L., Perel J.M., Peindl K.S., Hanusa B.H., Findling R.L., Rappaport D. (2001). Prevention of recurrent postpartum depression: A randomized clinical trial. *Journal of Clinical Psychiatry.* 62(2):82-86.

Yawn B.P., Bertram S., Kurland M., Wollan P.C. 2015. Repeated depression screening during the first postpartum year. *Annals of Family Medicine.* 13,(3): 228-234.

Resources

Postpartum Support International
6706 SW 54th Avenue
Portland, OR 97219
Office: (503) 894-9453
Support Helpline: (800) 944-4773
www.postpartum.net

Postpartum Support International (PSI) helps women get help as quickly as possible in all 50 states and in 49 foreign countries. PSI coordinators are trained to answer questions about postpartum depression, offer telephone support, and to listen for emergency situations. They also will recommend the nearest expert who can diagnose and treat postpartum psychiatric disorders.

To contact PSI, visit their website, www.postpartum.net. Click on "Get Help" and then click on the desired state or country. Or, call the helpline at 1-800-944-4773. Someone will answer your call live or return your call within 24 hours.

Academy of Breastfeeding Medicine
140 Huguenot Street, 3rd floor
New Rochelle, NY 10801
(800) 990-4ABM (USA toll-free)
www.bfmed.org

The Academy of Breastfeeding Medicine is a worldwide organization of physicians dedicated to the promotion, protection, and support of breastfeeding and human lactation. Their mission is to unite into one association members of the various medical specialties with this common purpose.

American Association of Family Practice Physicians

P.O. Box 11210
Shawnee Mission, KS 66207
(800) 274-2237 or (913) 906-6000
www.aafp.org/afp/topicModules/viewTopicModule.
htm?topicModuleId-16
This AAFP webpage features the best content from AAFP on labor, delivery, and postpartum issues and related topics, including breastfeeding, cesarean delivery, episiotomy, labor pain management, postpartum hemorrhage, preterm labor and birth, shoulder dystocia, umbilical cord blood storage, and vaginal delivery.

Depression and Bipolar Support Alliance (DBSA)

730 Franklin, Suite 501
Chicago, IL 60610
(312) 642-0049 or (800) 826-3632
www.dbsalliance.org
Formally known as the National Depressive and Manic-Depressive Association, the mission of the DBSA is to improve the lives of people living with mood disorders. DBSA reaches more than 1 million people each year. They offer information about depression and bipolar illness through their toll-free information and referral line and their website.

DOULAS International

35 East Wacker Drive, Suite 850
Chicago, IL 60601
(888) 788-DONA (3662) or (312) 224-2595
www.dona.org
Doulas are trained professionals who provide continuous physical, emotional, and informational support to the mother before, during, and just after birth. Doulas can also provide emotional and practical support during the postpartum period. Studies have shown that when doulas attend birth, labors are shorter with fewer complications, babies are healthier, and they breastfeed more easily.

Resources

Freedom from Fear
308 Seaview Avenue
State Island, NY 10305
(718) 351-1717
www.freedomfromfear.org
Freedom from Fear is a national not-for-profit mental health advocacy association founded in 1984. The mission of FFF is to aid and counsel individuals and their families who suffer from anxiety and depressive illnesses.

International OCD Foundation
P.O. Box 961029
Boston, MA 02196
(617) 973-5801
https://iocdf.org
The mission of the International OCD Foundation is to help all individuals with obsessive compulsive disorder (OCD) and related disorders to live full and productive lives. The foundation works to increase access to effective treatment, end the stigma associated with mental health issues, and foster a community for those affected by OCD and the professionals who treat them.

Marcé Society
P.O. Box 30853
London, W12 OXG
www.marcesociety.com
The Marcé Society is an international society for the understanding, prevention, and treatment of mental illness related to childbearing. The principal aim of the society is to promote, facilitate, and communicate information about research into all aspects of the mental health of women, their infants, and partners around the time of childbirth. This involves a broad range of research activities ranging from basic science through to health services research.

Massachusetts General Hospital
Center for Women's Mental Health
Perinatal and Reproductive Psychiatry Program
Simches Research Building
185 Cambridge Street, Suite 2200
Boston, MA 02114
www.womensmentalhealth.org
This hospital and treatment center in Boston, MA, has a very useful website. It also has a treatment center for perinatal psychiatric disorders. MGH also administers the National Pregnancy Registry for Atypical Antipsychotics.

Motherisk
Motherisk is a website maintained by The Hospital for Sick Children (Sick Kids). Sick Kids is a health care, teaching, and research center affiliated with the University of Toronto. Motherisk counselors talk to hundreds of women and their health care providers each day, providing guidance and support. Motherisk counselors are available Monday through Friday, from 9 A.M. to 5 P.M. EST.
(877) 327-4636 Alcohol and Substance
(800) 436-8477 Morning Sickness
(877) 439-2744 Motherisk Helpline
(416) 813-6780 Motherisk Helpline
http://motherisk.org/women/contactUs.jsp

National Alliance for the Mentally Ill (NAMI)
3803 North Fairfax Drive, Suite 100
Arlington, VA 22203
(703) 524-7600
www.nami.org
The National Alliance for the Mentally Ill (NAMI) is a nonprofit, grassroots, self-help, support and advocacy organization. It serves consumers, families, and friends of people with severe mental illnesses, such as schizophrenia, major depression, bipolar disorder, obsessive-compulsive disorder, and anxiety disorders.

National Institutes of Health
www.nlm.nih.gov/medlineplus/postpartumdepression.html
Produced by the National Library of Medicine, the world's largest medical library, NIH provides information about diseases, conditions, and wellness issues in language you can understand. The website also provides information on signing up for clinical trials.

National Institute of Mental Health
6001 Executive Boulevard
Rockville, MD 20852
www.nimh.nih.gov/health/publications/postpartum-depression-facts/index.shtml
This U.S. government website has information about psychiatric disorders with information and resources for consumers and clinicians.

National Pregnancy Registry for Atypical Antipsychotics
The National Pregnancy Registry for Atypical Antipyschotics is maintained by Massachusetts General Hospital in Boston. Participants in the registry, women 18 to 45, are monitored to determine the frequency of major malformations, such as heart defects, cleft lip, or neural tube defects, in infants exposed to atypical antipsychotics and antidepressants during pregnancy.
(866) 961-2388
E-mail: registry@womensmentalhealth.org.
www.womensmentalhealth.org

National Suicide Prevention Lifeline
www.suicidepreventionlifeline.org
(800) 273-TALK (8255)
The National Suicide Prevention Lifeline provides free and confidential emotional support to people in suicidal crisis or emotional distress. It operates twenty-four hours a day, seven days a week. Since its inception, the Lifeline has engaged in a variety of initiatives to improve crisis services and advance suicide prevention.

Postpartum Men
5835 College Avenue, Suite D3
Oakland, CA 4618
(415) 346-6719
www.postpartummen.com
Postpartum Men is a place for men with concerns about depression, anxiety, or other problems with mood after the birth of a child. It promotes self-help, provides important information for fathers, including a self-assessment for postpartum depression. The site hosts an online forum for dads to talk to each other, offers resources, gathers new information about men's experiences postpartum, and—most importantly—helps fathers to beat the baby blues.

Postpartum Progress
4920 Atlanta Highway, #316
Alpharetta, GA 30004
www.postartumprogress.org
Postpartum Progress is a unique, peer-to-peer organization that works to create an atmosphere in which women can recognize when they need help for maternal mental illness. The site helps them know that a community of thousands of other mothers stands beside them and behind them. Their website and blog provides good information in plain English. Postpartum Progress also promotes their Warrior Moms program through their website.

University of Arkansas
Mental Health Services
for Pregnant and Postpartum Women
4301 West Markham Street
Little Rock, AR 72205
(501) 686-7000
http://uamshealth.com/medicalservices/
behavioralmentalhealth/womensmentalhealth/
postpartumdepression
The website for UA Mental Health Services features resources for women's health. The hospital also offers a women's health clinic.

University of Miami Medical School
Women's Reproductive Mental Health Program
1400 N.W. 12th Avenue
Miami, FL 33136
General Information (305) 689-5511
Physician Referral (305) 689-5000
www.psychiatry.med.miami.edu
The University of Miami Miller School of Medicine Department of Psychiatry and Behavioral Sciences is committed to conducting research that deepens understanding of the development, pathophysiology, and prevention of psychiatric illness and the nature of human behavior. They apply this knowledge to the development and delivery of more effective, evidence-based treatments. They offer comprehensive treatment and consultation to their patients, families, and the community.

Glossary

adjustment disorder: a reaction to an external stress beyond what is considered typical.

agoraphobia: a symptom of anxiety in which you fear and often avoid places or situations that might cause you to panic and make you feel trapped, helpless, or embarrassed.

ambivalence: experiencing simultaneous and contradictory attitudes or feelings (such as attraction and repulsion) toward the baby.

androgen: any natural or synthetic compound, usually a steroid hormone, that stimulates or controls the development and maintenance of male characteristics.

anxiety disorders: several kinds of anxiety disorders can occur during pregnancy and postpartum. These disorders range from the excessive and uncontrollable anxiety of generalized anxiety disorder to the heart racing, short of breath episodes of panic attacks.

attunement: a mother's "knowing" her baby and his or her needs.

atypical antipsychotics: a group of antipsychotic drugs that tend to block receptors in the brain's dopamine pathways.

baby blues: refers to a brief time of temporary tearfulness, mood swings, fatigue, and perhaps irritability that typically only lasts one to two weeks.

benzodiazepines (BZD): sometimes called "benzos." These are a class of psychoactive drugs that enhance the effect of the neurotransmitter *gamma-aminobutyric acid (GABA)* at the GABA-AA receptor, resulting in sedative, sleep-inducing, antianxiety, anticonvulsant, and muscle relaxant properties.

143

bipolar disorder: characterized by fluctuating moods. There are episodes of depression at times and then there may be periods of excessive energy and grandiose thinking. Irritability, impulsivity, and poor judgment may also be a part of this disorder.

clinical trials: experiments done in clinical research. Research studies on human participants are designed to answer specific questions about biomedical or behavioral interventions, including new treatments and known interventions that warrant further study and comparison.

cognitive-behavioral therapy: therapy that emphasizes the influence of thinking on mood.

compulsions: a strong, usually irresistible impulse to perform an act, especially one that is irrational or contrary to one's will.

dopamine: a chemical found in the brain that acts as a neurotransmitter.

dysthymia: a chronic mild form of depression.

electroconvulsive therapy (ECT): a procedure to treat severe depression using electrical impulses briefly sent to the brain.

estrogen: a female sex hormone produced by the ovaries, adrenal glands, placenta, and fatty tissues.

GABA (gamma-aminobutyric acid): a biologically active substance found in the brain and other tissues; it is a neurotransmitter that inhibits activation of neurons.

generalized anxiety disorder (GAD): illness characterized by a persistent uncontrollable, unfounded worry, that affects most areas of a person's life.

group therapy: involves several patients meeting with one or more therapists in a group setting.

hypomania: an abnormal condition of extreme excitement, milder than mania but characterized by great optimism and overactivity.

interpersonal therapy: based on a relationship between a patient and a therapist. The basic premise is that there is a connection between one's mood disorder and the current interpersonal relationships in your life.

light therapy: therapeutic exposure to full-spectrum artificial light that simulates sunlight, used to treat various conditions, such as seasonal affective disorder.

mania: characterized by irrational excitement, occasionally violent behavior, and delusions.

manic-depressive disorder: *See* bipolar disorder.

MAOIs (monoamine oxidase inhibitors): refers to a category of antidepressant drugs that alleviate depression by stopping the monoamine oxidase enzyme from metabolizing neurotransmitters within the nervous system.

mood stabilizers: chemicals that are designed to balance the neurotransmitters in the brain for the benefit of controlling behavior and emotional states.

neurons: nerve cells that transmit information by electrical and chemical changes.

neurotransmitters: a chemical by which a nerve cell communicates with another nerve cell or with a muscle.

norepinephrine: substance that acts both as a neurotransmitter and hormone, secreted in the central nervous system, at the nerve endings of the sympathetic nervous system, and by the adrenal gland.

obsessions: a persistent idea or impulse that continually forces its way into consciousness, often associated with anxiety and mental illness.

obsessive compulsive disorder: repetitive intrusive thoughts and compulsions that are accompanied by feelings of guilt and shame.

panic disorder: a more extreme form of anxiety, marked by intense episodes of anxiety, usually accompanied by a fear of impending death.

perinatal: a more inclusive term, meaning "around delivery." This time period includes pregnancy and after delivery. Also called by some pre/post/partum.

peripartum onset: a term used to describe symptoms that occur during pregnancy or postpartum.

persistent depression: a chronic mild form of depression.

persistent depressive disorder: a chronic type of depression in which a person's moods are regularly low. Symptoms are not usually as severe as with major depression.

postpartum depression: a mood state marked by feelings of guilt, sadness, lack of enjoyment, fatigue, and problems in concentration. More severe symptoms may include thoughts of harming yourself or your baby.

postpartum psychosis: a state of confusion, agitation, being out of touch with reality, and having delusions and/or hallucinations. It is considered a psychiatric emergency because of the risk of harm to the baby or the mother. Postpartum psychosis usually develops in the first few days after delivery.

post-traumatic stress disorder (PTSD): a specific kind of anxiety disorder marked by re-experiencing a trauma such as a health event for the pregnant mother or fears about the fetus health, nightmares, and avoidance that does not lessen in intensity over time.

premature birth: birth of an infant after the period of viability but before full term.

progesterone: a female sex hormone produced by the ovaries.

prolactin: protein hormone secreted by the anterior portion of the pituitary gland that stimulates and maintains the secretion of milk in mammals.

psychotherapy: the treatment of psychological disorders or maladjustments by a professional technique, such as psychoanalysis, group therapy, or behavioral therapy.

relaxation therapy: using relaxation techniques to help promote calmness.

residency: the period during which a physician gets specialized clinical training.

schizophrenia: a psychiatric disorder marked by hallucinations and delusions as well as other symptoms.

selective serotonin reuptake inhibitors (SSRIs): antidepressants that prevent the reabsorption, or reuptake, of serotonin.

serotonin: a compound that occurs in the brain, intestines, and blood platelets and acts as a neurotransmitter, as well as inducing vasoconstriction and contraction of smooth muscle.

tricyclic antidepressants: a class of drugs used to treat depression and having a tricyclic chemical structure consisting of two benzene rings fused to opposite sides of a seven-member ring.

Index

147

Index

153

Index

symptoms, 47, 48
sexual abuse, 7, 29, 38, 61, 82
sexual desire decrease, 93
sexual problems, 93, 95
shame and embarrassment, 28, 68, 73
shortness of breath, 4, 45, 55, 56, 58
Sichel, Dr. Deborah, 69
Silencing the Self: Women and Depression, 29
single mothers, 124
sleeping problems, 19, 21, 26, 33, 37, 40, 41, 42, 48, 49, 53, 54, 62, 63, 66, 71, 93, 94, 97, 102, 106, 110, 121
Smith, R.N., Ann, 105
social commitments, 111
social environment, 34
social isolation, 6
social support, 84
social workers, 16, 79, 80, 81
    internships, 80
socializing techniques, 107
sociological stress, 29
spectrum of feelings, 46
startle response exaggeration, 63
stress, 5, 8, 30, 31, 78, 119
    hormones, 88, 90
    levels, 8
    management, 35
    reactions to, 51
    reduction, 121
    response, 18
substance abuse, 38
suicidal thoughts, 27, 29
suicide attempts, 27
suicide plan, 27
supplements, 77, 103
support groups, 105, 113
support system, 12, 78, 102, 120
supportive therapy, 102
sweating, 45, 58

T

tardive dyskinesia, 99
tearfulness, 3, 21, 91
testosterone, 90
thoughts of death, 27
thyroid gland, 30, 51, 90
tolerance of medication, 96
tranquilizers, 96
trauma, 4, 38, 51, 61, 63, 82
treatment options, with psychotherapy, 78
tremors/trembling, 93
tricyclic antidepressants, 94, 95
    side effects, 94, 95
Trintellix, 94

U

unrealistic expectations, 12
urination problems, 95

V

Valium, 96
valproic acid, 98
venlafaxine, 94
Viibyrd, 94
vilazodone, 94
violence, 29
Vistaril, 97
vortioxetine, 94

W

weaning baby, 36, 37
weight gain, 95, 99
weight loss, 30
Wellbutrin, Wellbutrin SR, Wellbutrin XL, 94
work commitments, 111
working women, 12

X

Xanax, 96

Z

ziprasidone, 98
Zoloft, 93
Zyprexa, 98

About the Author

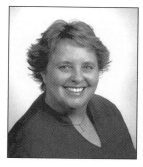

Linda Sebastian, A.R.N.P., has been an advanced nurse practitioner for thirty years. She specializes in women's mental health concerns, especially for pregnant and postpartum women. She is in private practice in Fort Myers, Florida.

As former director of the Women's Program at the Menninger Clinic in Topeka, Kansas, Ms. Sebastian was instrumental in developing the perinatal psychiatric disorders program and educated many health professionals about postpartum depression and anxiety. The Women's Program at Menninger was recognized nationally several times for its treatment of depression in women.

Ms. Sebastian received a master's degree in psychiatric nursing from Kansas University. She graduated from Wesley School of Nursing in Wichita, Kansas. She is the author of numerous professional journal articles, and has been a featured speaker in the United States and China.

Ms. Sebastian may be contacted through her website: **www.LindaSebastian.com**

Consumer Health Titles from Addicus Books

Visit our online catalog at www.AddicusBooks.com

To Order Books:
Visit us online at: www.AddicusBooks.com
Call toll free: (800) 888-4741

For discounts on bulk purchases, call our Special Sales
Department at (402) 330-7493.
Or e-mail us at: info@AddicusBooks.com

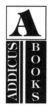

Addicus Books
P. O. Box 45327
Omaha, NE 68145

*Addicus Books is dedicated to publishing consumer health books
that comfort and educate.*

To order books from Addicus Books:

Please send:

_____ copies of _____

(Title of book)

at $ _____ each   TOTAL   _____

NE residents add 5% sales tax   _____

Shipping/Handling
$6.75 for first book
$1.10 for each additional book   _____

TOTAL ENCLOSED   _____

Name _____

Address _____

City _____ State _____ Zip _____

☐ Visa   ☐ Mastercard   ☐ AMEX   ☐ Discover

Credit card number _____

Expiration date _____

Four digit CVV number on back of card _____

Order by credit card or personal check.

To Order Books:
Visit us online at: www.AddicusBooks.com
Call toll free: (800) 888-4741

Addicus Books
P. O. Box 45327
Omaha, NE 68145

160